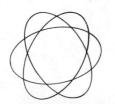

HOMEOPATHY
MEDICINE
OF THE
NEW MAN

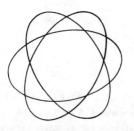

HOMEOPATHY
MEDICINE OF THE NEW MAN

George Vithoulkas

A FIRESIDE BOOK
Published by Simon & Schuster
New York   London   Toronto   Sydney   Tokyo   Singapore

Title Page: HOMEOPATHY
Typeface: CALEDONIA
Disk: BONNIE & WHITNEY

FIRESIDE
Simon & Schuster Building
Rockefeller Center
1230 Avenue of the Americas
New York, New York 10020

Published in 1987 by Prentice Hall Press
First Fireside Edition 1992
Originally published by Arco Publishing, Inc.

FIRESIDE and colophon are trademarks
of Simon & Schuster Inc.
Manufactured in the United States of America

20 19 18 17 16 15 14 13 12

Library of Congress Cataloging-in-Publication Data
Vithoulkas, George
Homeopathy.

Bibliography: p. 146
Includes index.
1. Homeopathy—Popular works.   I.   Title
RX76.V57   615'.532   77-29272

ISBN 0-671-76328-8

Contents

Foreword

We are living in one of the most exciting periods in human history. Virtually every aspect of human life is undergoing radical conceptual change—science, politics, economics, ecology, theater, music, etc. Such change even extends to the field of medicine. The objectified, materialistic view of the world is widening to include the energetic plane of existence. The concept of the whole man is replacing the previously fragmented view of the patient as a diagnostic entity. In the fields of holistic health, nutrition, acupuncture, etc., increasing trust is being placed on the healing forces of the individual, rather than on drugs.

This book by George Vithoulkas represents the cutting edge of this movement in the field of medicine. Step by step, it takes us through uncanny discoveries which have led to the most effective curative system known to mankind. In contrast to the somewhat vague mysticism which inevitably characterizes the early, stumbling steps towards true holistic medicine, Vithoulkas' book demonstrates convincingly that homeopathy is a systematic science which correctly applies the laws of nature to stimulate the healing energies of the human being.

1

The respect that I have for the work of Vithoulkas can best be illustrated by briefly describing my own story. From a young age, enamored of the "white coat" image of medicine, I decided to become a doctor. I finally succeeded, graduating from Stanford Medical School, where I was steeped in the most solidly materialistic of medical science.

After completing my training, I contemplated going into private practice, but my idealistic image of what medicine should be left me disappointed and frustrated with what I had learned. I turned to the holistic fields of nutrition, herbal medicine, acupuncture, chiropractics, and polarity massage, but nowhere could I find a method that was systematic enough to deal with the deep chronic diseases which are the challenge of every physician. Finally, I received training in homeopathy and opened a private practice in Northern California.

The results I received through homeopathy were gratifying, but there were still many, many cases which I myself knew I had inadequate knowledge to treat. It was at this time that I met George Vithoulkas. His analysis of some of my cases taught me quickly that in the hands of a true Master, homeopathy holds the answer for the vast majority of chronic disease sufferers.

The degree of respect I developed for Vithoulkas' knowledge of homeopathy is best measured by the fact that I finally closed my practice in California and left my own teaching responsibilities in order to study with him full-time in Athens, Greece. I have never regretted this decision, for it has brought about the possibility of my delivering the precise, natural cure to my patients which is the goal of every conscientious physician the world over.

It may seem too good to be true, but humankind's centuries of searching for a non-toxic, truly curative medicine have finally come to completion in the homeopathic system. The challenge we now face is to create a professional school in which the highest standard of homeopathic medicine can be taught with the dedicated strictness which is necessary.

In this landmark work, George Vithoulkas convincingly and concisely describes the basic foundations upon which this seemingly miraculous method is built.

BILL GRAY, M.D.

I

Coming of the New Age

In recent years, a profound revolution in thinking about health and disease has emerged. Beginning with a thoughtful and well-informed public seeking more effective means of dealing with chronic diseases, it has come to influence the medical profession itself as well as policy-makers in government.

It is difficult to trace exactly where the roots of this line of thinking began in modern times. Historically, it stretches back to Hippocrates and before, but with the advent of technology and the strictly materialistic worldview, it became lost for a time. Its resurgence has been influenced by the growth of psychology, the Esalen-inspired view of the whole man, the re-awakening of spiritual and mystical consciousness, and even the awareness of ecology. It is a revolution inspired by the high level of education achieved in modern times.

Arising from this trend are a variety of clinics, classes, seminars, publications, and businesses loosely described as the "holistic health" movement. The basic concept is that each of us is an integrated whole. We are not fragmented into separate parts each carrying a specific ailment or diagnostic category. We cannot be divided by any belief, lifestyle, relationship, or therapy without violating fundamental universal laws. Each of us is a unique individual, whole and complete, functioning as a totality in relation to the universe surrounding us. All states of health or disease must be viewed in this context. To the extent that we deviate from this perspective, we experience disharmony and dis-ease. Conversely, the more we live within this principle, the more we enjoy a balanced state of harmony and vitality.

A second basic tenet of the holistic approach is that the most effective, indeed the *only*, way to cure illness is to increase the health of the afflicted person. There is a fundamental recognition that all living beings are animated by a "vital force" (to be discussed in considerable detail later) which when disturbed leads to sickness, and when activated leads to health. This force (called by the Chinese "Chi," and the Hindus "prana") has yet to be scientifically isolated, observed, or measured, but each of us is aware of it working within us.

We all have made the observation that some of our friends enjoy a higher degree of vitality than others. Each of us experiences fluctuations in energy from hour to hour and day to day; we tend to ascribe these changes to stresses, diet, sleep, etc. But, whatever the apparent "cause," the *experience* is one of increasing or decreasing vital energy.

A holistic practitioner, then, helps the "client" to identify the various aspects of his life which tend to enhance the natural processes, and which aspects tend to oppose them. Thus, the primary responsibility for the recovery of his health is placed upon the shoulders of the client himself.

In this context, symptoms are seen as attempts by the body to heal or to signal distress, and they are respected as such—in marked contrast to the standard medical approach in which symptoms are viewed as disturbances to be suppressed.

Let me discuss some of the principal holistic practices in order to clarify the setting in which homeopathy is to be seen.

The first holistic approach to gain widespread approval by public common sense was nutrition. First popularized by author Adelle Davis in the 1950s, good nutrition was quickly recognized as being fundamental to proper health. As awareness of the necessity for a proper balance of nutrients grew, the public began consulting their doctors for advice on diet and vitamins—only to discover that they knew more in this area than their physicians and that no medical school in the United States taught nutrition. This was the first major step in the gradual dissolution of the mystique surrounding medicine.

With time, the nutrition movement grew beyond the fad stage inaugurated by Adelle Davis and returned to the type of nutrition upon which the human race has actually evolved. But two principles were emphasized: the provision of proper nutrients (primarily through grains, seeds, nuts, vegetables, and fruits), and the detoxification of the body by various means. Thus, the vital force is sustained by a proper balance of nutrients and simultaneously liberated from the burden of toxicity.

To nutrition and detoxification was added recognition of a third basic bodily need—exercise. Throughout evolution, until the last century or so, exercise has been a fundamental aspect of daily existence. In the last several years there has been a virtual explosion of interest in exercise, not only as a therapy, but also as a form of self-discovery and sheer enjoyment. America, known as a nation of armchair sportsmen, suddenly became a nation of joggers, tennis buffs, cyclists, soccer players, and swimmers.

Nutrition and exercise are fine for maintaining health once achieved, but what of those in need of therapy? In answer to this, acupuncture was suddenly "discovered" and embraced in the United States. Acupuncture is a technique in which needles are carefully and systematically placed in the skin in strategic locations so as to stimulate the flow of the vital force along channels or pathways known as meridians. In this system, illness is viewed as an obstruction or imbalance in the flow of the vital force, which can be re-balanced by the insertion of needles.

At the same time, a variety of other techniques designed to do essentially the same thing were either rediscovered or popularized: polarity massage, Lomi massage, reflexology, various movement and posture techniques, Hatha Yoga, chiropractics, osteopathy, and others. With the availability of all of these techniques, people with chronic diseases gradually came to believe that the body's own natural healing processes could be nurtured unobstructed, and rebalanced with definite benefit—and without the toxicity of drugs, radiation, or surgery.

Unfortunately, initially high expectations held by chronic disease sufferers were frustrated in the end. Although the new techniques provided some degree of comfort, *cure* seemed to be no closer than with traditional medicine. To maintain benefit, the patient must continue with frequent treatments, often with diminishing or transient results. The new approaches were still merely *techniques*, without fundamental insight into the origins of chronic diseases and without solid principles on which to base therapy.

It is in this context that large numbers of people have turned to the highly sophisticated science of homeopathy.

In my experience of twenty years of practice, it is perhaps the most effective natural medicine against acute and chronic illness existing today. At last, the epitome of holistic medicine has been reached, and actual cure has become a reality rather than merely a dream.

II

Samuel Hahnemann and the Law of Similars

"The physician's highest and only calling is to restore health to the sick, which is called Healing." Samuel Hahnemann.[1]

Homeopathy is a very highly systematic method of powerfully stimulating the body's vital force to cure illness. It is based on a few simple but profoundly insightful principles of Nature which are contrary to commonly held beliefs.

[1] S. Hahnemann, *Organon of the Art of Healing* (sixth American edition; Boericke and Tafel, Philadelphia, 1917; translated from the fifth German edition by C. Wesselhoeft, M.D.), p. 13.

Sometimes in the footnotes and throughout the bibliography no publisher is indicated for a work mentioned. This means that the work is a standard textbook of homeopathy and that it exists in different editions and sometimes in different translations.

Quotations from Samuel Hahnemann's *Organon*, for instance, have been taken either from the translation of C. Wesselhoeft, M.D., which he has entitled *Organon of the Art of Healing*, or that of W. Boericke, M.D., entitled *Organon of Medicine*.

"Organon" is a Greek word which signifies "the means."

In all its ramifications, homeopathy is far too sophisticated a discipline to be learned in a few seminars, or by reading this book. The principles are simple in concept, but difficult to fully comprehend, and they require years of intensive training and experience to apply—as many, or more, years as in a standard medical school.

To properly introduce homeopathy, we must go back 170 years and examine perhaps the most remarkable story in medical history, all encompassed in the life of one man. With time, I am certain that this man will rank as one of the greats in history, alongside such giants of discovery as Einstein, Newton, and Hippocrates. Like these men, his insights have radically and permanently altered our perceptions of not only health and disease, but also the nature of existence itself. For this reason, we shall trace the life and thought of this man in some detail as a means of explaining and clarifying the basic principles of homeopathy.

In 1810, a book entitled *Organon of the Art of Healing* was published in Torgaou, a small town in Germany. Its author, Samuel Hahnemann, was an extremely prominent physician and medical author of the time, so that the appearance of another book under his name generated automatic interest. However, once the book was read, the European medical community was thrown into an uproar, for it introduced an entirely new and radical system of medicine, one fundamentally opposed to the traditional medicine of the time.

Hahnemann called his new medicine homeopathy, a word taken from the Greek *omeos*, meaning "similar," and *pathos*, meaning "suffering." Thus, homeopathy means "to treat with something that produces an effect similar to the suffering." In his book, Hahnemann laid out the laws and principles of his science, gathered empirically over a period of twenty years.

Briefly, Hahnemann claimed and showed that:

1. A medical cure is brought about in accordance with certain laws of healing that are in nature.
2. Nobody can cure outside these laws.
3. There are no diseases as such, but only diseased individuals.
4. An illness is always dynamic by nature, so the remedy too must therefore be in a dynamic state if it is to cure.
5. The patient needs only one particular remedy and no other at any given stage of his illness. Unless that certain remedy is found, he is not cured but at best the condition is only temporarily relieved.

Because of its dramatically curative results, homeopathy was soon to win widespread approval throughout Europe and the world; but when Hahnemann's work was first published it met with the most bitter opposition from doctors who were still prescribing blood-letting, cathartics, and diaphoretics. Hahnemann was not discouraged. He was a brilliant individual and, as such, was used to being misunderstood.

His first biographer, Thomas Bradford, describes how Hahnemann's father used to lock his son up with what he called "thinking exercises"[2]—problems the boy was required to solve himself. In this way, Hahnemann learned to develop the use of intuition and insight, and to come to know the limitations of intellectual logic.

Clearly, Hahnemann was precocious at virtually everything he attempted. When he was twelve, his teacher had him teaching Greek to the other students. He put himself

[2] Thomas Lindsley Bradford, M.D., *Life and Letters of Dr. Samuel Hahnemann* (Philadelphia: Boericke and Tafel, 1895).

through university studies of chemistry and medicine by translating English books into German. He qualified as a physician from the University of Leipzig in 1779, and soon after began publishing a series of works on medicine and chemistry. In 1791, his research in chemistry earned him election to the Academy of Science in Mayence. His *Apothecary's Lexicon* became a standard textbook for the time, and he was chosen from all the physicians in Germany to standardize the German *Pharmacopoeia*.

Soon after graduating from medical school, Hahnemann married and had children. He now had a family, and his reputation in the fields of both chemistry and medicine was firmly established, yet he was dissatisfied. Hahnemann dropped the practice of medicine, much to the dismay of his colleagues and friends. As he wrote to a friend, "It was agony for me to walk always in darkness, when I had to heal the sick, and to prescribe, according to such or such an hypothesis concerning diseases, substances which owed their place in the *Materia Medica* to an arbitrary decision. . . . Soon after my marriage, I renounced the practice of medicine, that I might no longer incur the risk of doing injury, and I engaged exclusively in chemistry, and in literary occupations."

After he had become a father, when disease threatened his "beloved children," he still was not swayed. In fact, as he wrote to the same friend, "My scruples redoubled when I saw that I could afford them no certain relief." He continued translating medical works as a meager means of supporting his family. He could have made a very comfortable living practicing medicine, but he preferred poverty to the necessity of conforming to a system "whose errors and uncertainties disgusted me."

Hahnemann's active mind nevertheless remained curious, open, and systematic. He relentlessly probed into the basic issues of health and disease. It was in this frame of mind that he stumbled onto the first fundamental principle of homeopathy. He was translating the *Materia Medica* (a compendium of the actions of therapeutic agents), written by Professor Cullen of London University. Cullen devoted twenty pages of his book to the therapeutic indications of Peruvian Bark (a source of what is known today as quinine), attributing its success in the treatment of malarias to the fact that it was bitter. Hahnemann was so dissatisfied with this explanation that he did something very extraordinary: He took a series of doses of Peruvian Bark himself! This was an action entirely unprecedented in the medical world of his time. It is not known to this day what prompted him to do such a thing, but his experiment led to an entirely new era of medicine. He describes the result as follows:

I took by way of experiment, twice a day, four drachms of good China. My feet, finger ends, etc., at first became cold; I grew languid and drowsy; then my heart began to palpitate, and my pulse grew hard and small; intolerable anxiety, trembling, prostration throughout all my limbs; then pulsation in the head, redness of my cheeks, thirst, and, in short, all these symptoms, which are ordinarily characteristic of intermittent fever, made their appearance, one after the other, yet without the peculiar chilly, shivering rigor.

Briefly, even those symptoms which are of regular occurrence and especially characteristic—as the stupidity of mind, the kind of rigidity in all the limbs, but, above all the numb, disagreeable sensation, which seems to have its seat in the periosteum, over every bone in the body—all these make their appearance. This paroxysm lasted two or three hours each time, and recurred if I repeated this dose, not otherwise; I discontinued it, and was in good health.[3]

[3] T. L. Bradford, *op. cit.*, pp. 36–37.

Imagine the astounding revelation that struck Hahnemann as a result of this experiment! The standard medical assumption had always been that if the body produces a symptom, a medicine must be given to relieve that symptom. This was so deeply ingrained that it had almost become an automatic reflex in the mind of doctor and patient. But here, in his own personal experience, Hahnemann found that a drug which was known to be curative in malaria actually produces those very symptoms when given to a healthy person!

Many would simply have ignored such an observation as a mere exception. Hahnemann, however, was a true empirical scientist. To him, the observation itself was what counted—regardless of whether it fit neatly into current dogmas or not. He accepted the observation and went on to make further experiments which further proved this "chance" observation as a fact of Nature: *A substance which produces symptoms in a healthy person cures those symptoms in a sick person.*

This discovery, as well as the fact that he was already very well known, attracted to Hahnemann a number of physicians who, like himself, were looking for the truth. They all started to experiment upon themselves by taking different drugs. They continued for six years and kept scrupulously detailed records of the symptoms produced upon each of them by every drug they had taken.

During this time Hahnemann, who had access to a vast medical library and was fluent in Latin, Greek, Arabic, English, and French, compiled an exhaustive list of accidental poisonings recorded by different doctors in different countries through centuries of medical history. The symptoms produced by poisons and those produced by experiments done upon Hahnemann's physician friends were gathered together in detailed volumes. Hahnemann and his colleagues recognized in these symptom pictures the identical symptomatologies of many illnesses for which medical science had in vain been seeking cures. These medicines were then tried on patients who manifested similar symptoms, and the amazing discovery was made that the drugs actually cured so-called "incurable" diseases when prescribed according to this principle. According to the law he had discovered, Hahnemann saw that every drug must necessarily cure the set of symptoms it produces in a healthy human organism.

The process by which Hahnemann and his colleagues experimentally produced the symptoms of a substance upon their healthy organisms he called "proving." Orthodox medicine (which homeopaths term "allopathic," from *allo* meaning "other") also has its process of proving drugs, but with the very important difference that it experiments upon animals.

Animals do not possess the power of speech. They cannot report the subleties of alterations in mood or the different types of pain which can be described by human experimental subjects. In addition, the physiology of animals is considerably different from that of the human being. Hahnemann perceived clearly that any therapeutic system based upon animal experimentation must necessarily be limited. To construct a valid therapy, experimentation must be done within the same realms of physiology and awareness as the medicines will be called upon to act therapeutically. This principle is merely common sense, yet it was absolutely revolutionary in Hahnemann's time.

After several years of experimentation, Hahnemann returned to the practice of medicine, but now he was practicing homeopathy. During a consultation, Hahnemann first noted down all the patient's symptoms, mental and physical; he then sought a homeopathic medicine that had produced similar symptoms in himself or one of his associates (or which had been observed from an accidental poisoning). Prescribing in this manner, he achieved a rate of cure which was truly remarkable. Moreover, these cures tended to be speedy and permanent—sometimes even after a single dose of medicine!

Hahnemann's rationale for the homeopathic principle, known today as the Law of Similars, is explained in Aphorism 19 of the *Organon*:

Now, as diseases are nothing more than alterations in the state of health of the healthy individual which express themselves by morbid [i.e., disease-producing] signs, and the cure is also only possible by a change to the healthy condition of the state of health of the diseased individual, it is very evident that medicines could never cure diseases if they did not possess the power of altering man's state of health which depends on sensations and functions; indeed, that their curative power must be owing solely to this power they possess of altering man's state of health.

Although he had so clearly grasped and formulated this principal law of homeopathy, Hahnemann did not feel that he had discovered it. He quotes a number of people who, he thought, either stated it or hinted at it long before he did. Hippocrates, for instance, stated this law several times in his teachings, referring to two methods of cure: by "contraries" and by "similarities." Boulduc wrote long before Hahnemann's time that rhubarb's purgative quality was the reason why it cured diarrhea; another writer named Betharding said that the herb senna cures colic because it produces a similar effect on the healthy. And Stahl, a contemporary of Hahnemann, wrote that "the rule accepted in medicine to cure by contraries is entirely wrong; on the contrary diseases vanish and are cured by means of medicines capable of producing a similar affection."[4]

Going back in history as far as the ancient Jewish Bible, we find the Mekilta stating, in effect, that whereas man heals with contrary remedies, God heals with similars! "Come and see, the healing of the Holy One, blessed be He, is not like the healing of Man. Man does not heal with the same thing with which he wounds, but he wounds with a knife and heals with a plaster. The Holy One, blessed be He, however is not so, but He heals with the very same thing with which he smites."[5]

Although others had grasped the principle, Hahnemann's genius went a large step further. He had the perceptiveness to reason that if the Law of Similars is a basic truth, then we should be able to identify the curative properties of substances by systematically testing them on normal people. It was this systematic method which was the first of his many major contributions to medical thought.

[4] S. Hahnemann, *Organon of the Art of Healing*, p. 46.
[5] Quoted from MEKILTA DE—RABBI ISHMAEL, translated by J. Z. Lauterbach, The Jewish Publication Society of America, Phila., p. 239.

III

Preparation of Homeopathic Medicines

Once Hahnemann felt he had proven enough remedies, he began prescribing them in the accepted dosages of the time; but although the patient was invariably cured, the drug often caused such a severe initial aggravation of symptoms that patients and doctors alike became alarmed. Such aggravation was to be expected since the drug itself was producing symptoms similar to those of the patient. Moreover, Hahnemann wanted to test some of the drugs in common use at that time—drugs such as mercury and arsenic; but, of course, he could not give such toxic substances to healthy people.

So he reduced the dose to one-tenth of its customary amount. The patient was still cured but the aggravation, though lighter, remained. This was not good enough. Hahnemann diluted the medicine still further, each time prescribing only one-tenth of the previous dose, and presently reached a dilution that was completely ineffective because there was essentially no more medicine left in it.

The advantages of simple dilution were clearly very limited. If the medicine was not strong enough to aggravate the symptoms, it was too weak to bring about a cure. The future of homeopathy seemed to be on shaky grounds, indeed.

Precisely at this most critical juncture, Hahnemann made another amazing discovery. To this day, it is not exactly known how Hahnemann came upon the procedure; most likely, it arose from his knowledge of chemistry and alchemy. In any case, he simply submitted each dilution to a series of vigorous shakes (or "succussions," as he called them) and discovered that progressive dilutions were then not only less toxic but also more potent![6]

Hahnemann had found a solution to a problem that had occupied medical men throughout history. He had beaten the problem of the "side effect" of drugs!

We shall presently offer certain theories as to why this happens, but we know from observation that it does. Hahnemann says that the efficacy of a remedy thus processed is increased because "the powers, which are, as it were, hidden and dormant in the crude drug, are developed and roused into activity to an incredible degree."

Hahnemann first considered that distilled water, alcohol, and lactose (milk sugar) were medicinally inert, so he diluted the medicines in these substances. If the remedy were soluble in water or alcohol, he mixed one part of the substance with ninety-nine parts of the liquid and submitted the mixture to one hundred vigorous succussions. This dynamized solution he called the "first centesimal potency." Then he mixed one part of this first potency with ninety-nine parts of water or alcohol and

---

[6] At this point, the author would like to invite the experience and papers of all scientists who could explain this event, either by experiment or by existing literature.

again succussed the dilution one hundred times to produce the second centesimal potency. The third step in the process, of course, diluted the original substance to one part in a million, the fourth step to one part in a hundred million, and so on. He repeated this up to thirty times and apparently did not go beyond that himself, although modern homeopaths use potencies to the *hundred thousandth centesimal* and beyond!

The implications of this discovery are staggering. A substance shaken and diluted to a dilution of 1 in 100,000 parts, even to a total of 60 zeros and more, still acts to cure disease, quickly and permanently, and without side effects!

Clearly this phenomenon cannot be explained by ordinary chemical mechanisms. The dilutions are so astronomical that not even one molecule of the original medicine is left! And yet the actual clinical results demonstrate beyond a doubt that *some* influence remains—an influence which is powerful enough to cure even deep chronic diseases. In Aphorism 209, Hahnemann writes:

The homeopathic system of medicine develops, for its special use, to a hitherto unheard-of degree, the inner medicinal powers of the crude substances by means of a process peculiar to it and which has hitherto never been tried, whereby only they all become immeasurably and penetratingly efficacious and remedial.

What Hahnemann had discovered is that there lies hidden in every substance in Nature some inner life. We can mobilize and use this "force" if we know how to process the substance correctly.

Science has shown that, when it is possible to *reduce* a substance to its molecular state and to isolate a molecule, this particular molecule exhibits an automatic, incessant mobility, known as "Brownian Movement." Every atom and molecule is composed of high degrees of energy, and the particles contained within atoms move at speeds often approaching that of light. Everyone today is aware that tremendous energy can be released by the fission of fusion of atoms. From these observations, it is clear that hidden within the apparently solid material substances of our world are vast amounts of energy lying dormant.

Somehow, the repeated dilutions and succussions of a homeopathic medicine release a great curative energy which is inherent in the substance. In each instance above, we discover that energy is released by the proper method. We do not know the relationship, if any, between these phenomena, but there is objective proof that they exist: Brownian Movement is observed by looking through the microscope at minute particles suspended in water; modern quantum physics measures with great precision the energies and speeds of motion of subatomic particles; and nuclear explosions demonstrate the energy contained in matter. In homeopathy we witness the amazing cures that the potentized remedy can bring about.

In this connection, we are struck by something which the famed healer Paracelsus wrote centuries ago: "The Quintessence is that which is extracted from a substance. . . . After it has been cleansed of all impurities and its perishable parts, and refined to the highest degree, it attains extraordinary powers and perfections. . . . In it there is great purity, and it is because of this purity that it has the virtue to cleanse the body."[7]

As we have seen in the holistic health field—not to mention the impact of Einstein and modern quantum physics —we have gone beyond the concept of Nineteenth Century

[7] Karl Sudhoff and Wilhelm Matthiessen, eds., *Paracelsus, Samtliche Werke*, part 1, Vol. II, pp. 186–187 (translated by the author).

materialism and accepted quite easily the idea that all matter is, in fact, energy, and that this energy can be released and even harnessed. The true miracle is that in homeopathy it has been harnessed for the cure of disease.

IV

The Vital Force

"We may regard matter as being constituted by the regions of space in which the field is extremely intense. . . . There is no place in this new kind of physics both for the field and matter, for the field is the only reality." Albert Einstein

Insight into the fact that all matter is permeated with energy which can be liberated for the purpose of curing disease eventually led Hahnemann to the true understanding of the nature of disease. He had the kind of mind that proceeded only from facts obtained from research, inquiry, and experiment. He never accepted any concept that was incompatible with the results of experiment and observation.

Now, two facts struck him: firstly, that remedies greatly diluted could only cure if they were homeopathically potentized, that is, energized through succussion; and seconly, that once they were so potentized they contained no detectable material trace of the original substance. It followed therefore that their curative effect was not a material affair but that it involved some other factor—energy. He concluded that the succussions must transmit some of the energy of the original substance to the neutral matter in which it was diluted. We see examples of such transmission in our daily lives: plastic transmitting static electricity to paper if rubbed against it; or electricity, an invisible force, being stored in batteries which are themselves material. He probably realized that he had gone beyond matter and was working in the domain of energy.

From all this, a chain of logical conclusions necessarily followed. Since the remedy was in fact *dynamic* and not material, the level of disorder upon which it worked must belong to the same order of being: so the illness was a derangement primarily on a dynamic plane. But what exactly did that mean? Hahnemann concluded that it was simply a derangement in the life force in man. The transition from life to death takes no time at all, is not measurable in time, not gradual; yet it is the most radical transition there is. It ends all activity of the body and decomposition follows. This dynamic force which makes the difference between a corpse and a human being Hahnemann called the "vital force." In Aphorism 9 he describes its qualities:

In the healthy condition of man, the spiritual vital force (autocracy), the dynamism that animates the material body (organism), rules with unbounded sway, and retains all the parts of the organism in admirable, harmonious, vital operation, as regards both sensations and functions, so that our indwelling, reason-gifted mind can freely employ this living, healthy instrument for the higher purposes of our existence.

The mind must be extremely free and perceptive to comprehend so clearly something which is neither visible nor material. Nobody can deny that some force holds the universe together simply because this force is invisible or immeasurable. All of us experience this vital force in our daily lives when under stress—a change in climate, travel, change in diet, unusual exertion, a grief, a momentary illness. In all of these instances, we observe in ourselves a resiliency, a flexibility, an ability to adapt to circumstances. As this ability is most dramatically evident only in living things, we call it vital force.

Today we have at our disposal the means of recognizing a force by its qualities alone and that is how we recognize the existence of such things as magnetism, electricity, the force of gravity, and so on. The usual definition of electricity is that it is a movement of electrons, but we know nothing about the force which makes that movement possible. The very essence of force or energy has always eluded us and we have never been able to perceive it or comprehend its nature through the senses. Similarly, the vital force which animates the body is not something we can experience directly; its presence can only be recognized through its qualities.

James Tyler Kent, one of the most illustrious American physicians of the Nineteenth Century, describes some of its qualities in his *Lectures on Homeopathic Philosophy*:

1. It is endowed with formative intelligence, i.e., it intelligently operates and forms the economy of the human organism.
2. It is constructive; it keeps the body continuously constructed and reconstructed. But when the opposite is true, when the vital force from any cause withdraws from the body, we see that the forces that are in the body being turned loose are destructive.
3. It is subject to changes; in other words, it may be flowing in order or disorder, may be sick or normal.
4. It dominates and controls the body it occupies.
5. It has adaptation. That the individual has an adaptation to

his environment is not questioned, but what is it that adapts itself to environment? The dead body cannot. When we reason we see that the vital force adapts itself to surroundings, and thus the human body is kept in a state of order, in the cold or in the heat, in the wet and damp, and under all circumstances.[8]

Another proof of the existence of this vital force is the fact that when the disturbed organism of a patient is properly tuned through the administration of the right homeopathic remedy, the patient not only experiences the alleviation of symptoms, but also has the feeling that life once again is harmoniously flowing through him. Finally, after centuries of stumbling and experimenting, we have a system of medicine that not only recognizes the presence of the healing powers of the body and of Nature, the vital force, but actually bases its entire system upon the stimulation of that force. At last, principles were found by which we can work with, rather than against, the vital force—a true ecology of medicine.

[8] James Tyler Kent, M.D., *Lectures on Homeopathic Philosophy* (Calcutta: Sett Dey & Co. 1961), p. 69.

V

The Dynamic or
Subtle Plane

Once the basis of health and healing was understood, Hahnemann applied his genius to the question of disease. In Aphorism 11 he writes: "When a person falls ill, it is only this spiritual, self-acting (automatic) vital force, everywhere present in his organism, that is primarily deranged by the *dynamic* influence upon it of a morbific agent inimical to life" (emphasis mine).

Here we see clearly that Hahnemann went far beyond his time, and was even in advance of us today, in stating that not only the disease but also its cause is dynamic. In other words, it is not the microbes or the virus or the bacteria, nor even their virulent poisons on the biochemical level that cause disease, but rather their intimate nature, their vital force, their very "soul." And that is something *dynamic*.

Furthermore, these vibrating, pulsating, living inner malevolent or morbific (meaning "harmful" or "destructive") agents can only affect organisms that are susceptible

28

to them, and can only affect them on a dynamic energy level. If illness were a question of bacteria and their numbers, those most exposed would be the first to be affected. But we all know that this is not the case. There are people everywhere who are exposed to contagious diseases and do not catch them. People sleep in the same bed with victims of tuberculosis or severe staphylococcal infection and are never affected. Correspondingly, there are others who live in the most healthy environment and take great care with diet, rest, exercise, etc., and still contract all kinds of contagious infections.

Disease comes about only when two conditions are fulfilled: the presence of an external morbific agent and the patient's own susceptibility. It is not merely the result of exposure to a number of microbic invaders. That is why an epidemic never hits everybody in a particular area.

All allopathic physicians are taught that susceptibility is a major factor in the production of disease. This fact is taught, but it is subsequently ignored as the overwhelming emphasis of medical training and practice focuses exclusively upon the theory of viral or microbic transmission of disease. It is readily acknowledged that people are protected from microbial attack by "antibodies," but no further inquiry is made into precisely what triggers off the production of antibodies. Again, why is it that this happens to certain people and not to others?

The great American homeopath of the Nineteenth Century, J. T. Kent, again writes:

They will tell you that the bacillus is the cause of tuberculosis. But if man had not been susceptible to the bacillus he could not have been affected by it. . . . The bacteria are results of the disease. . . . the microscopical little fellows are not the disease cause, but they come after. . . . They are the outcome of the disease, are present wherever the disease is, and by the

microscope it has been discovered that every pathological result has its corresponding bacteria. The Old School considered
these the cause . . . but the cause is much more subtle than
anything that can be shown by a microscope.[9]

So we can clearly see that both susceptibility and a destructive agent are necessary for the appearance of disease.
It is interesting to note here that the theory of "allergic
conditions"—to which orthodox medicine subscribes—
fully supports this. It states that even an infinitesimal
quantity of a substance can sometimes bring about such
violent reactions in someone susceptible to it that the
suffering is unbearable, and in rare instances even fatal.
This happens because his susceptibility to the substance
has laid him open to its effects. Since in their daily practice
allopathic doctors observe infinitesimally small amounts
of substance causing disease, one wonders why they do not
accept that an equally small dose of remedy can cure it,
particularly since a homeopathic remedy is selected precisely because it has the closest possible affinity with the
patient's disorder, and he is therefore most sensitive to it.

If we wish to seek a scientific explanation for the action
of infinitesimal homeopathic doses, we will find it in the
law of Maupercius, the Eighteenth Century French mathe-
matician, who said: "The quantity of action necessary to
effect any change in nature is the least possible; according
to this principle the decisive amount is always a minimum,
an infinitesimal."[10]

This principle can be seen in action all around us. How
much warmth is required to unleash the incredible growth
potential in a seed? How much energy from the sun is
needed in order to nourish a single flower? Think of how

[9] J. T. Kent, M.D., *op. cit.*, p. 22.
[10] Quoted in Dr. H. A. Roberts, *Principles and Art of Cure by
Homeopathy* (England: Health Science Press, 1962), p. 119.

sensitive the instruments must be which measure cosmic rays from the sun—yet cosmic rays unleash tremendous forces in the vast weather changes occurring during sunspot cycles.

Today more than ever, mental shock is recognized as the sole exciting cause of a series of diseases. If we accept in these cases the dynamic disturbance caused by a thought or an emotion, why is it difficult to accept that the initial disturbance lies always on an energy level which can be affected also by the inherent vibrating energy of the bacteria or the microbe?

The conviction that disease is caused by bacteria is probably one of our greatest illusions. All therapeutic research today is based on this tenet; it has produced a continuous wave of new products, new medicines, at a quite incalculable cost in time, effort, health, and money. But it is based on a wrong assumption and directed towards the wrong target. Many people argue that orthodox medicine, as the result of research, has impressively reduced the death-rate all over the world, but if we look around us we can see that the incidence of mental and emotional illness has increased proportionately. We will later speak of the relationship between these two phenomena.

In homeopathic practice, the contrary is the case. It is not at all a question of killing bacteria but of bringing the whole human organism into a state where it is impossible for bacteria to thrive on it—in other words, to reduce the patient's susceptibility.

To summarize, then, what we have said so far:

1. A patient is cured only if he is given that medicine that can produce in a healthy organism symptoms most similar to his own.
2. A disease is not just the malfunction of some organ but,

first of all, a disturbance of the vital force that is responsible for the functioning of the whole organism.

3. Medicines cannot penetrate the physical organism to reach and to act upon the vital force unless they are in a dynamic, energized state.

4. The cause of disease must be sought on a dynamic plane and not on a physical-chemical plane.

VI

Predisposition to Disease

Now let us return to the question asked by all sufferers of chronic disease: What is the *real* cause? How did this arise in my case? And what does this mean for my treatment?

As we have said, Hahnemann attracted a great many medical men who helped him in his work of proving the different remedies and recording the provings. His cures won him countless admirers. Students flocked from all over the world to study under him. But success also made him many bitter enemies. One of these, a prominent Leipzig publisher, looked for someone to write a book against homeopathy and found a certain Dr. J. H. Robi, who passed on this task to his pupil, Constantine Hering. Hering accordingly set about investigating homeopathy and tried to collect material which would discredit it. Instead, he was rapidly convinced of its inherent truth and became devoted to Hahnemann and homeopathy. He collected, classified, and published all existing information on the action which drugs exert on human beings. His monumental *Materia Medica* runs into twelve large volumes and has become a fundamental reference book in homeopathy.

One rarely fails to find in it any symptom, mental or physical, which has been produced by the proving of a remedy—no matter how strange: a fever that only comes between six and eight o'clock in the evening; a chronic headache that comes on alternate days and lasts from ten in the morning till three in the afternoon; a vertigo that appears only when the patient is lying down with eyes closed; an irrational fear that if one goes to sleep one will never wake up; depression and sadness that emerge only in twilight; irrational fears—of cancer, heart disease, death, or insanity; a suicidal impulse to jump from a great height; a neuralgic pain that appears only once a week; an excruciating sciatic pain that comes every fourth day; a rheumatic pain that strikes only between two and four in the morning; an asthmatic attack that comes at midnight. . . .

By this time the resources at the homeopath's disposal— his knowledge of the science and its laws, his techniques of preparing the remedies—were much greater, considerably more refined and accurate. Seeing this, Hahnemann applied himself, from 1816 onwards, with his customary order and penetration to the understanding of disease itself.

He observed that diseases are of two general classes. The first are usually self-limited and brief; in Aphorism 72, Hahnemann defines them: "Such affections usually run their course within a brief period of variable duration, and are called *acute* diseases." *Chronic* diseases, the second class of diseases, are more insidious and destructive in the long-run. They represent an entirely different problem both for the vital force of the patient and for the homeopath. Hahnemann continues: "The second class embraces diseases which often seem trifling and imperceptible in the beginning; but which, in a manner peculiar to themselves, act deleteriously upon the living organism, dynamically deranging the latter, and insidiously undermining its health to such a degree, that the automatic energy of the vital force, designed for the preservation of life, can only make imperfect and ineffectual resistance to these diseases in their beginning, as well as during their progress. Unable to extinguish them without assistance, the vital force is powerless to prevent their growth or its own gradual deterioration, resulting in the final destruction of the organism."

For Hahnemann, the cure of acute diseases presented no great problem. Simply find that substance which produces similar symptoms in a healthy organism, and the cure is rapid and complete. But chronic diseases were a different matter. To comprehend how Hahnemann met this challenge, we must go back and follow his discoveries step by step.

From 1810 to 1816, the six years after he published the *Organon*, he was inundated with pupils and patients from all over the world. He kept a complete record of every case, and noticed that, although the great majority of complaints were cleared up, many patients subsequently returned with a new complaint, or a relapse of the old one. It was in Hahnemann's nature to ask why and to probe until he had found the answer. In his *Chronic Diseases*, he writes:

Whence then this . . . unfavorable result of the continued treatment of the . . . chronic diseases even by Homeopathy? What was the reason [for] the thousands of unsuccessful endeavors to heal . . . diseases of a chronic nature so that lasting health might result? Might this be caused, perhaps, by the still too small number of Homeopathic remedies that have so far been proved as to their pure action? . . . Even the new additions of proved valuable medicines, increasing from year to year, have not advanced the healing of chronic diseases by a single step, while acute diseases are not only passably removed, by means of a correct application of Homeopathic remedies but with the assistance of the never-resting preservative vital in our organism, find a speedy and complete cure.

Hahnemann saw time and again chronic diseases removed homeopathically only to return in a more or less varied form and with new symptoms. He saw that the homeopathic physician, presented with a chronic case, "has not only to combat the disease presented before his eyes, . . . but that he has always to encounter some separate fragment of a more deep-seated original disease. . . . He, therefore, must first find out as far as possible the whole extent of all the accidents and symptoms belonging to the unknown primitive malady before he can hope to discover one or more medicines which may homeopathically cover the whole of the original disease."

To Hahnemann, it gradually became clear that such chronic conditions cannot be cured by the vital force alone, nor by any manipulation of diet or life habits. He then launched into exhaustive inquiries of all such chronic cases to see if any common denominator could be found to explain the deep and invisible weakness which predisposed to their chronic condition—a weakness which Hahnemann termed "miasm." By 1827, when Hahnemann had studied this problem for about twelve years, he became convinced that he had found the common denominator. His conclusion was based upon two related observations.

Hahnemann describes the first observation in the following passage: "I had come thus far in my investigations and observations with such . . . patients, when I discovered, even in the beginning, that the obstacle to the cure of many cases . . . seemed very often to lie in a former eruption of *itch*, which was not infrequently confessed; and the beginning of all the subsequent sufferings usually dated from that time." In patients who at first could not recall any such itchy skin eruption, Hahnemann persistently inquired in even further detail into every stage in the life of the patient: "After careful inquiry it usually turned out that little traces of it (small pustules of itch, herpes, etc.) had showed themselves with them from time to time, even if but rarely, as an indubitable sign of a former infection of this kind."[11]

This initial clue as to the basis of miasmatic predispositions to chronic disease was further confirmed by a second type of observation made by many physicians of that time. The following are a few of the case histories Hahnemann quotes in his *Chronic Diseases*, which he gathered from many different physicians:

A boy of 13 years having suffered from his childhood with *Tinea Capitis* [known today as "ringworm of the scalp"] had his mother remove it for him, but he became very sick within eight or ten days, suffering with asthma, violent pains in the limbs, back and knee, which were not relieved until an eruption of *Itch* broke out over his whole body a month later (Pelargus, ((Storch)) *Obs. clin. Jahrg.* 1722, p. 435).

Tinea Capitis in a little girl was driven away by purgatives and other medicines, but the child was attacked with oppression of the chest, cough, and great lassitude. It was not until she stopped taking the medicines and the *Tinea* broke out again, that she recovered her cheerfulness and this, indeed, quickly (Perlargus, *Breslauer Sammlung v. Jahre*, 1727, p. 293).

11 This and other quotes in this section on chronic diseases are from *The Chronic Diseases* (Calcutta: C. Ringer and Co.), translated by Prof. Louis H. Tafel, pp. 19–22.

A 3-year old girl had the *Itch*, for several weeks; when this was driven out by an ointment she was seized the next day by a suffocating catarrh with snoring, and with numbness and coldness of the whole body, from which she did not recover until the *Itch* re-appeared (Suffocating Catarrh, Ehrenfr. Hagendorn, *hist. med. phys. Cent. P. hist.* 8, 9).

A boy of 5 years suffered for a long time from *Itch*, and when this was driven away by a salve it left behind a severe melancholy with a cough (Riedlin, the father, *Obs. Cent. II, obs.* 90, Augsburg, 1691).

A girl of twelve years had the *Itch* with which she had frequently suffered, driven away from the skin by an ointment, when she was seized with an acute fever with suffocative catarrh, asthma, and swelling, and afterward with pleurisy. Six days afterward, having taken an internal medicine containing sulphur, the *Itch* again appeared and all the ailments, excepting the swelling, disappeared; but after twenty-four days the *Itch* again dried up, which was followed by a new inflammation in the chest with pleurisy and vomiting (*Pelargus, Obs. clin. Jahrg.,* 1723, p. 15).

A girl of 9 years with the *Tinea Capitis* had it driven away, when she was seized with a lingering fever, a general swelling and dyspnea; when the *Tinea* broke out again she recovered (Hagendorn, *Recueil d'observ. de Med. Tom. III,* p. 308).

From *Itch* expelled by external application there arose amaurosis, which passed away when the eruption re-appeared on the skin (Amaurosis, Northof, *Diss. de scabie,* Gotting., 1792, p. 10).

A man who had driven off a frequently occurring eruption of *Itch* with an ointment fell into epileptic convulsions, which disappeared again when the eruption reappeared on the skin (Epilepsy, J.C. Carl in *Act. Nat. Cur. V., obs.* 16).

Two children were freed from epilepsy by the breaking out of humid *Tinea*, but the epilepsy returned when the *Tinea* was incautiously driven off (Tulpius, *obs. lib. I., Cap.* 8).

From these cases two facts emerge. First, in a person with a deep chronic disease tendency, when a skin eruption is merely suppressed instead of being properly cured, it brings about serious disturbances in inner organs; and second, all the organs of the body are the interrelated parts of but one organism and therefore influence each other mutually.

There is no such thing then as a "local disease"; one may use this expression only to mean that a particular part of the body is more especially affected, but not that one organ suffers independently of the others. Modern orthodox medicine subscribes more and more to this view, that there are no diseases but only individuals who are ill —but only with lip-service. For instance, in the case of a patient suffering from asthma, constipation, and rheumatic pains, today's allopathic physician will prescribe three different medicines—one for each ailment (and each one probably a combination of several drugs as well)—whereas the homeopath would prescribe a single remedy to cure the single disease which is showing itself in three aspects.

To return to Hahnemann and his inquiry into the origin of chronic diseases, the numerous examples he mentions show us clearly the connection between skin diseases and internal disturbances. He also observed that whenever he brought about a real cure, the skin disorder from which the patient suffered in the past reappeared during treatment and whenever the patient was relieved of the internal trouble.

This fundamental miasm underlying the majority of chronic diseases Hahnemann termed *Psora*. He viewed it as a fundamental weakness further aggravated by suppressive treatments which merely remove the symptom without curing the predisposition.

Man's efforts to get rid of suffering merely resulted in continuous suppression of diseases throughout the ages. Except by some lucky chance or otherwise, very few people ever received the right treatment, and the continued suppression of symptoms created damaging weaknesses in internal organs. These weaknesses were transmitted from one generation to the next, according to Hahnemann's investigations, which included whenever possible interviews with the ancestors of chronic disease patients. Children inherit from each parent particular sensitivities in particular organs, and the resulting disorder in the child is either an accurate copy of one parent's disorder, or a compounding of disorders inherited from both parents.

Hahnemann had noticed that, whereas nature tries to keep the disorder as far as possible from man's vital organs—as far as possible from his center, as it were—when the vital defensive resources become critically diminished, the disease proceeds to more internal organs.

Not only are the physical impediments of the parents involved, but other factors as well: mental disposition of the parents at the time of conception, hardships they have suffered physically and mentally, their habitual diet, the degree of toxicity of their bodies (children conceived when the parents were heavily under the influence of alcohol or drugs are particularly affected), even the magnetic conditions of the atmosphere and the degree of atmospheric pollution, radioactivity, and so on. All of these, as well as any disturbing influence during pregnancy, will affect the sensitivity of the unborn child.

This, briefly, is the beginning of Hahnemann's theory

of the basic cause of diseases. "The psoric miasm," he writes, "is the most ancient, most universal, most destructive, and yet most misapprehended miasm, which for many thousands of years has disfigured and tortured mankind, and which during the last centuries has become the mother of thousands of incredibly various, acute, and chronic (non-venereal) diseases. . . ."

The concept of the "miasm" may seem too simple, too pat. It may seem too easy to lay the origin of all chronic diseases to such a single simple source—particularly something as seemingly insignificant as a skin eruption. Doctors reading this may balk at the idea that the vast advances in therapy over the centuries have largely resulted in suppression of the vital force, and therefore a worsening of the chronic disease state of mankind. But before you dismiss the concept, remember that Hahnemann was a recognized, pioneering, medical genius who applied himself painstakingly to the question for twelve years. It also is true that solutions to the most difficult problems are generally very simple, and usually come from an unexpected quarter. Finally, as always, the final proof lies in the fact that Hahnemann's insight has led to the most consistently dramatic and permanent cures of chronic diseases ever seen.

Hahnemann was very careful to distinguish between venereal and non-venereal diseases. The reason for this was that his studies of ancient history led him to the conclusion that venereal diseases were a much more recent phenomenon than Psora. As we have seen, Hahnemann took great pains to prove the transmissive "miasmatic" character of skin eruptions. Syphilis was a simpler matter: he did not have to convince anybody of its ability to be transmitted from generation to generation. It was common knowledge at that time that syphilis could not really be eradicated, but rather that its effects were transmitted through successive generations.

It is a very frequent observation in homeopathic practice that the Syphilitic miasm is grafted onto an organism which has already been weakened by the Psoric miasm. In Aphorism 206 of the *Organon*, Hahnemann writes, "When a physician is called to treat what he supposes to be an inveterate case of syphilis, he will usually find that it is principally complicated with psora, because this miasm (the psoric) is by far the most frequent and fundamental cause of chronic diseases. . . ."

In this situation, the homeopath is faced with a difficult and delicate problem. *Two* specific miasmatic predispositions are present at the same time. The homeopath must be able to discern which symptoms belong to the Syphilitic miasm, and remove this layer first. Only then will the symptom complex representing the Psoric miasm become clear. Each miasm is represented by a set of symptoms. Therefore, the homeopath must recognize among the totality of symptoms those complexes which belong to each miasm. Obviously, this is a painstaking process, demanding extraordinary skill and knowledge on the part of the prescriber and a great deal of patience on the part of the patient.

Hahnemann also identified a third miasm, which he labelled the Sycotic miasm. This arises from a certain type of gonorrhea which has the peculiarity of developing warts in its secondary stage. "The miasm of the other common gonorrheas," Hahnemann writes, "seems not to penetrate the whole organism, but only locally stimulate the urinary organs."

The homeopath confronted with a case in which all three miasms are present can remove them one by one— not simultaneously. Remedies prescribed must follow each other in a particular sequence depending upon the prominence of a particular miasm at any particular moment in time. This demands the homeopath's constant attention, continuous study, and careful re-evaluation of the symptoms appearing during various phases of treatment; only their correct assessment will enable the prescriber to choose the right remedy in the right dose at the right time.

Unfortunately, in our time the task is even greater than it was in Hahnemann's time. There are in fact many more than three miasms. Modern homeopathic experience identifies a wide variety of influences which can engraft upon the constitution predispositions which are transmitted from generation to generation.

A common source of miasms are severe diseases such as cancer or tuberculosis. It is well known that such ailments run in families, and homeopaths are also able to identify specific symptom complexes found in subsequent generations which are related to these diseases without necessarily resulting in the specific diseases themselves.

Another source of miasms are the vaccinations and powerful drugs commonly prescribed by allopathic doctors. These can create such disturbance in the vital force that the patient is left with a chronically weakened state. Specific iatrogenic miasms which are commonly seen in homeopathic practice arise from smallpox vaccinations, cortisone, major tranquilizers, antibiotics, and other powerful drugs.

Because of all of these influences, it is not uncommon these days to encounter patients suffering from five or six miasmatic layers. In addition to the Psoric miasm, there may exist the sycotic miasm, plus a "smallpox vaccine" miasm, a "penicillin miasm," a "cortisone miasm," etc. For a homeopath, a case of this type presents the most tragic, disheartening, and frustrating kind of challenge to his skills. To peel off each miasmatic layer in succession, even assuming that correct prescriptions are made each time, can take many years of painstaking and patient effort.

One word of clarification, so as not to touch off a panic among most of my readers: Merely because someone has taken a drug does not mean that he or she suffers from that miasm. Only a relatively small number of people who take such drugs for a long time, or who get gonorrhea or syphilis for that matter, actually acquire the corresponding miasm. Nevertheless, even this small percentage of patients presents a serious problem in a society in which chronic diseases are the major health issue.

VII

The Homeopathic
Interview

We may have, by now, some idea of the enormous task
the homeopath assumes when he agrees to take our case.
In addition, he must answer questions like: "Can you
cure me?" "How long will it take?" "What must I do to
cooperate?" Today, every patient knows the name which
orthodox medicine has given to the prominent symptoms
of his or her trouble. He must also know, from the beginning, that no true homeopath prescribes according to the
name of a disease: each case is new, each has its own particular symptoms, mental and physical. Each individual is
unique. A homeopath who bases his prescription on the
name of the disease instead of on the patient is no true
homeopath and should not be trusted.

How does a homeopath look to a patient? What is it
like to experience a homeopathic interview? To begin
with, the literature in the waiting room will emphasize
natural approaches to medicine, and there will likely be
far fewer patients waiting than you will find in the office

45

of an allopath. This is simply because the length of each visit is considerably longer. Indeed, if you are not the first patient of the day, you may wait long past your own scheduled time, for the interview, as you will discover, is painstakingly individualized, and therefore nearly impossible to schedule by the clock.

During the interview, you might feel slightly self-conscious. It may seem that the homeopath is gently scrutinizing your every mannerism. But you quickly realize that this is not a process of passing judgment, but merely of interested observation. You soon get the idea he or she is as much or more interested in *you* as in your ailment.

In contrast to the allopathic doctor who rarely, if ever, turns to a book during consultation, the homeopath is surrounded by gigantic well-worn books to which he constantly refers as you describe particular symptoms, all the while writing incessantly in the chart. He may even request that you speak more slowly so that he can get the exact phrasing of your words!

If you are unfamiliar with these stylistic differences, you may have a sense of wonder at all this, a sense that will likely be reinforced when the homeopath, after listening at length to everything you can think of to say, launches into a long series of the most unusual questions, ranging widely into all aspects of your life. Are you warmblooded or do you usually feel chilly? Intolerant to dry or wet weather? Do you have any fears (of dogs, of the dark, of death, of closed places, of heights)? Are you anxious, and if so, over what kinds of things (your health, other people)? Are you unusually neat or sloppy? How are you affected by music? Are your complaints mostly on one side of your body—which side? Do you have any particularly strong cravings or aversions for specific foods? How do you sleep? What position do you sleep in? Do you stick your feet out from under the covers? All these questions and more may be asked. It may seem momentarily like psychoanalysis, except that the homeopath does not challenge or probe deeply into your answers, but simply notes them in your own phrasing and moves on.

At the conclusion of the interview, the homeopath may well require time for private study of your case in order to go into all the details with his books before he prescribes a remedy. You will likely leave the office with your mind awhirl with many details, wondering if you have answered his questions fully and correctly, since many will have involved subtleties about yourself you had never thought about—perhaps never *would* have thought about. Invariably, patients later return reporting a change in some of their answers after observing themselves more closely for awhile. But, as often, the homeopath will have anticipated them through his knowledge of the totality of symptoms of the remedy he has prescribed for you. This may lead you to conclude that the homeopath knows you better than you do yourself.

Hahnemann knew the complexities of human nature and the difficulties confronting the homeopath in trying to question a patient about his symptoms. In Aphorism 96 he writes: "It is worthy of remark that the temperament of patients is often abnormally affected; so that some, particularly hypochondriacs, and other sensitive and intolerant persons, are apt to represent their complaints in too strong a light, and to define them by exaggerated expressions, hoping thereby to induce the physician to redouble his efforts."

And in Aphorism 97: "But there are persons of another kind of temperament, who withhold many complaints from the physician, partly from false modesty, timidity or bashfulness; and who state their case in obscure terms, and who consider many of their symptoms as too insignificant to mention."

He went still further. He compiled a list of more than one hundred questions which the doctor should ask the patient in taking a case. This gives the reader some idea of the accuracy and care required in taking a case, and the time involved.

Take, as an example, the following case from the notebook of J. T. Kent. It deals with a lupus erythematosus growth of the nose; this diagnosis alone would be sufficient for any allopathic doctor to begin treatment (pessimistically, since there is no allopathic "cure" for this disease), whereas for Kent, a homeopath, we see how much information was needed to complete the cure:

Mr. H. C. M. was a married man, 28 years old when he appeared for treatment.

Oct. 1, 1903. Nose had a lupus growth across it, resembling a large red saddle. Malaria of nine months' duration five years ago. Checked by doctor with quinine. Irritable. Memory good. Sleeps reclining on back; inclination to place arms above head. Dreams depressing, latter part of night. Respiration slow. Heart pulse 60. Appetite and thirst small. Rheumatic pains in R. ankle, occasionally in shoulders. Steady pains in small of back. No pains intense. Agg. in winter, amel. in summer: itching and rheumatism. Skin dry; itching on cheeks and nose, and in winter on ears. Spots became hard, lumpy then red and very itchy; similar itching on head and in rectum. Has never had pimples nor boils. Used to have warts—burnt off. Feet always cold. Hair falling out. Tonsillitis recurrent. Perspiration copious from exertion. Urine light and yellow, frequent and copious. Rectal evacuation costive, daily, in morning. Sensitive to cold, not to heat. In childhood was sensitive to heat but always had cold feet. Urination frequent, difficult, urine nearly white, following the drinking of two glasses of beer when overheated ten years ago. Considers this the beginning of kidney-trouble and skin disorder. Nausea, riding in cars or on elevators. Psor. cm.

Nov. 7. Stomach—empty sensation. Itching over entire body. Rheumatism in joints; shoulder, wrists, elbows. Anus—moisture; itching. Kidney-region pain. Feet cold. Sensitive to cold. Psor. cm.

Dec. 16. Cold feet and sensitive to cold. No new symptoms.

March 4, 1904. Lupus has not broken out much this winter. Anus—moisture. Tired and languid; wants to recline. Constipation. Respiration sighing. Psor. cm.

April 23 and July 6. Psor. mm. Chief symptoms during this period were rheumatic pain in ankles, sensitiveness to cold, nausea riding on cars, hair dropping out, and moisture about anus.

Oct. 1 (about). Headache frontal. Stomach sour. Nose—lupus visible on crest and side of nose. Nausea, riding on elevated road cured by Psor.

Nov. 9 and Dec. 23. Sulphur. 10m.

Feb. 15. Pains in small of back. Pain in region of spleen. Headache frontal. Catarrh of nose. Slow to answer. Sleeps with covers over head.

Here the record ceases. The patient has remained cured many years.[12]

It would be no exaggeration here to say that love is needed. However, taking the case is only the first part of the picture, for the prescriber must then set about finding the remedy. To do so he must go through his books and study the provings of different drugs until he finds the one whose symptoms are the most similar to those of the patient. It often takes hours before the prescriber can say that he has found the right remedy for a chronic condition. In homeopathy, there are no ready-made formulas. Each case requires its own particular medicine, and no

[12] J. T. Kent, M.D., *Lesser Writings* (Calcutta: Sett Day and Co., 1958), pp. 411–412.

other potentized remedy will have any significant effect at all.

Considering all the difficulties involved in taking and prescribing for a chronic case, as well as the knowledge of miasms and the remedies themselves, it is very difficult for a conscientious homeopath to either promise a cure or define the time needed. And in any case it is an unscrupulous practitioner who promises a cure in whatever ailment. Generally, it seems the one who promises least will accomplish the most.

As a very gross rule, one can say that it will take a month of treatment for every year the patient has suffered. For instance, if the patient had the ailment for eight years, it will take approximately eight months to cure him. This is not an absolute rule. Often the length of time may be much shorter, and in other cases longer.

If a patient's case is very simple, it may be cleared within one consultation only, but in complicated cases, especially in those who have been taking allopathic drugs for several months or years, the process of really curing is a long and arduous one for both the patient and the homeopath. Finally, a lot will depend on the prescriber's skill and knowledge of homeopathy.

VIII

A Sample Case:
Influenza

The choice of the correct homeopathic medicine is not a simple one. One does not prescribe on a reflex basis: remedy A for a cold, remedy F for arthritis, remedy X for cancer, etc. Instead, each prescription must be highly individualized to the specific symptoms manifested by each patient, regardless of the formal diagnosis.

Of a group of ten patients having exactly the same disease, a homeopath may prescribe ten different remedies. Conversely, the same remedy is commonly prescribed to a variety of patients all suffering from different disorders.

Often, the decision of which remedy to give is based upon fairly subtle differences. The homeopath must be a very astute observer, very familiar with human nature, systematic, and thorough.

To provide an example of the subtleties of homeopathic prescribing, let us imagine an influenza epidemic. Throughout a typical day, a homeopathic prescriber may see several cases and prescribe different remedies in each case.

Influenza, being a dramatic acute ailment, is actually quite easy for homeopathic prescribing. Compared to usual dilemmas facing a homeopath, the differentiation between possible remedies in influenza is quite clear.

Virtually everyone is familiar with the common symptoms of influenza. Usually, it attacks with a fairly sudden onset. The patient develops a high fever, prostration, and usually headache and muscle aches. Most patients complain of sore throat, swollen lymph nodes, perhaps a runny nose, and later a cough. Sometimes there is nausea, vomiting, and diarrhea. These are the common symptoms by which the allopathic diagnosis "influenza" is made. However, as the following excerpts from Douglas M. Borland's monograph, *Influenzas*, demonstrates, there are many types of influenzas, each requiring different remedies. Herein we will consider only a handful of the many which could be presented—just a sample to provide you with a concept of the individualizing detail which leads to the correct prescription.

Gelsemium Sempervirens (Yellow Jasmine)

Gelsemium is somewhat slow in onset, and produces primarily a feeling of intense weariness. The patients are very dull and tired, look heavy, and are heavy-eyed and sleepy; not wanting to be disturbed but to be left in peace, and yet—the first outstanding symptom—if they have been excited at all, they spend an entirely sleepless night, in spite of their apparently dull, toxic state.

The patient is definitely congested, the face slightly flushed —rather a dull kind of flush—the eyes a little injected, the lips a little dusky; the skin generally is a little dusky, and the surface is definitely moist—hot and sticky.

Another Gelsemium symptom is that with the hot, sticky sensation, the patients have a very unstable heat reaction.

They feel hot and sticky, and yet have the sensation of little shivers of cold up and down their backs—not actual shivering attacks but small trickles of cold, just as if somebody ran a cold hand, or spilt a little cold water, down their back.

With their general torpor, Gelsemium influenza patients always have a certain amount of tremulousness, their hands become unsteady much more quickly than you would expect from the severity of their illness; they are definitely shaky when they lift a cup to try and drink. Frequently linked with the shakiness is a feeling of instability, and very often a sensation of falling. They feel as if they are falling out of bed, particularly when they are half asleep; they wake with a sudden jerk and feel as if they have fallen out of bed.

As one would expect with anyone in this toxic state, the Gelsemium patient does not want to make any effort at all; discomforts of every kind are aggravated by moving. With their unstable circulation they are definitely sensitive to cold draughts, which make them shiver.

As a rule, their mouths are intensely dry and the lips very dry; very often dry and cracked, or dry with a certain amount of dried secretion on them. The patients complain of an unpleasant taste, and there is frequently a sensation of burning in the tongue. The tongue itself usually has a yellowish coating—though, sometimes, it is quite red and dry.

Gelsemium influenzas always include a very unpleasant, severe headache. Typically, there is a feeling of intense pain in the occipital region, spreading down into the neck with a sensation of stiffness in the cervical muscles; and, as it is a congestive headache, it is usually throbbing in character.

The patient is most comfortable when keeping perfectly still, propped up with pillows, so that the head is raised without the patient making any effort. With these headaches, the patients often complain of a sensation of dizziness, particularly on any movement.

There is another type of headache sometimes met with in Gelsemium. Again, it is congestive in character, but the sensation is much more a feeling of tightness—as if there were a tight band round the head, just above the ears from the occiput right forward to the frontal region. This, also, is very much aggravated by lying with the head low.

Peculiarly, these patients often find relief from their congestive headaches by passing a fairly large quantity of urine.

In nearly all Gelsemium influenzas there is a sensation of general aching soreness, an aching soreness in the muscles. This is worth remembering; there are other drugs which have similar pains but are much more deep-seated than the Gelsemium pains.

Now for a few details of actual local disturbances.

Most Gelsemium patients have that appearance of intense heaviness of the eyelids that is associated with this dull toxic condition. But there is also a good deal of sensitiveness of the eyes themselves, a good deal of congestion, a definite sensitiveness to light, probably a good deal of lachrymation and general congestive engorgement.

There is an apparent contradiction here: despite this occular sensitiveness, occasionally a Gelsemium patient becomes scared in the dark and insists on having a light.

These patients get very definite acute coryza, with a fluid, watery discharge, accompanied by very violent sneezing and a feeling of intense fullness and pressure just about the root of the nose. It is not uncommon in Gelsemium influenza— where there is this feeling of blockage at the root of the nose —to find a story of epistaxis on forcible clearing of the nose. This, again, is worth remembering, for certain Mercurius cases tend to run in the same way.

With their acute coryzas, Gelsemium patients, despite a general hot stickiness, very often complain of very cold extremities. (This appears to be a contradiction, and might mislead you when you consider the general heat of the typical Gelsemium patient.)

As a rule, in Gelsemium influenzas, there is no very marked localised tonsillitis, but much more a generalised, puffy, red, congested throat. There may be a certain amount of enlargement of the tonsils, but it is not the spotty throat that some of the other drugs have.

In spite of the absence of acutely localised symptoms there is often acute pain on swallowing. Swallowing may be actually difficult—with a feeling of constriction or of a lump in the throat—and it is much more difficult when the patients take cold fluids than warm; this is unexpected, considering the dryness of their mouths.

Associated with these conditions of nose and throat, Gelsemium influenzas quite frequently have an involvement of the ears. But, in spite of what is recorded in the *Materia Medica*, I have not observed the acute stabbing pains that are described under Gelsemium; and, where I have tried to clear up such pains with Gelsemium, I have not had any success.

Gelsemium is given as one of the drugs that has stabbing pains into the ear on swallowing; in my experience, it has not been effective. Gelsemium does get a good deal of roaring in the ears, a feeling of blockage and obstruction and you very often get dullness of hearing, and giddiness; but I have not seen acute earaches respond to Gelsemium.

Quite frequently there is an extension downwards, with involvement of the larynx and loss of voice. Associated with the laryngitis, there is liable to be an intensely croupy cough which is almost convulsive in character, coming in spasms and associated with very intense dyspnea.

Typical Gelsemium patients, despite their sweatiness and dryness of mouth, are not usually very thirsty. Occasionally a patient is intensely thirsty, but the typical one is not.

They hardly ever have an appetite—they do not want anything at all. They very often complain of a horrible empty sensation in the region of their chest, often near the heart. This sometimes spreads down into the epigastric region, and they may describe it as an empty feeling; but it is not really a sensation of hunger, and is not associated with any desire for food.

Associated with the digestive system, Gelsemium patients often have a definitely yellowish tinge, and actual jaundice may develop. Again, the patient quite frequently develops very definite acute abdominal irritation accompanied by diarrhea. Usually, the stool is very loose and yellowish but not particularly offensive.

There is quite often a story of intense feeling of weakness in the rectum—an incontinence, or a feeling of prolapse—after the bowels have acted; and there is sometimes a definite prolapse associated with the diarrhea.

BAPTISIA (Wild Indigo)

Baptisia runs very closely to Gelsemium in symptomatology. Personally, I look at Baptisia as Gelsemium exaggerated, more intense.

In contrast to Gelsemium patients, Baptisia patients are definitely more dusky. They give you the impression that their faces are a little puffy and swollen; their eyes are heavy, but with a congested, besotted look rather than the drooping lids of Gelsemium; and lip congestion, present in Gelsemium, makes Baptisia lips rather blue.

Mentally, Baptisia patients are more toxic than Gelsemium patients; they are less on the spot; they are confused, finding it difficult to concentrate on what they are doing. They grow a little confused as to the sensation of their body; they may feel that their legs are not quite where they thought they were. Their arms may have definite disturbed sensations; some patients feel their arms are detached and they are trying to re-attach them, others say their arms are numb.

Associated with this is the general Baptisia confusion. The patients themselves are not quite clear why they are there, where they are, what they are talking about or trying to discuss; and they are not quite clear whether there is somebody else talking to them, somebody else in the bed. They are simply more fuddled than Gelsemium patients.

As you would expect with the slightly more intense toxemia, all the local conditions are definitely worse. The tongue is definitely dirtier—the typical Baptisia tongue is in a pretty foul state. In the early stages it usually has a central coating of yellow, brown or black with a dusky red margin all round.

The patient's breath is always foul. With this very foul mouth, there tends to be a lot of ropy, tough saliva which is apt to dribble out of the corner of the mouth when the patient is half asleep. In consequence, the lips tend to crack and become very foul, and may actually bleed. . . .

The Baptisia patient sweats a lot, but the sweat, in contrast to the somewhat sourish odour of Gelsemium, is definitely offensive. This is true of anything in connection with Baptisia; it is all offensive. . . .

In Baptisia, it is much more commonly the right ear and the right mastoid region which is involved. If a mastoid does occur, the prognosis is very serious indeed. Thrombosis occurs very early—and I mean astonishingly quickly—and the prognosis becomes correspondingly worse.

In a Baptisia influenza with obvious mastoid developing—tenderness and slight blush over the mastoid region—it is astonishing how the case alters completely within two or three hours of giving Baptisia. The patient, from being obviously toxic—all the signs of starting meningeal irritation are developing—is equally obviously recovering, as a result of even the first dose of Baptisia.

In contrast with Gelsemium, Baptisia patients are always thirsty. They have a constant desire for water, but if they take much at a time it often produces a sensation of nausea. Taking a little at a time, they are all right, but their thirst is always one of their troublesome features. . . .

Baptisia patients always have intense aching pains all over. Any part they press is painful and tender; they also have acute pains in their joints, a feeling as if they were sprained or had been bruised; moving is very painful.

BRYONIA ALBA (Wild Hops)

The typical Bryonia influenza develops, like the Gelsemium case, over a period of six to twelve hours. And the appearance of Bryonia patients is not unlike that of Gelsemium patients. They give the impression of being rather dull, heavy, slightly congested, with a rather puffy face.

Although they are definitely heavy looking, they do not have the sleepy appearance that you find in Gelsemium, nor yet the besotted look of the Baptisia patient—something between the two.

Mentally, as stated, Gelsemium patients are dull, sleepy, heavy and do not want to be disturbed. Bryonia patients are also definitely dull and do not want to be disturbed—but if they are disturbed they are irritable. Irritability is always cropping up in Bryonia patients. They do not want to speak, and do not want to be spoken to. They do not want to answer because speaking annoys them, not because they are too tired to do so.

As a rule, Bryonia influenzas are very depressed; they are despondent and not a little anxious as to what is happening to them; they feel they are ill and are worried about their condition.

To their worry about their impending illness they add a very definite anxiety about their business. They talk about it; if they become more toxic, they are apt to dream about it, and it is an underlying thought in the back of their minds throughout their illness.

It is also typical of Bryonia influenzas that the patients are difficult to please. They are very liable to ask for something and refuse it when it comes. They want a drink, and, when it comes, do not want it. Or, they may ask for a fruit juice drink and, when that comes, say they would much rather have had a drink of plain cold water—they are very difficult to satisfy.

Typically, they have a good deal of generalised, aching pain. They will tell you that it hurts them to move, and yet, very often, Bryonia patients are constantly on the move. They are restless and uncomfortable, and move about in spite of the fact that the movement increases their pain.

Get hold of this fact very clearly, because it is so definitely laid down in the text-books that Bryonia patients are aggravated by motion. Apparently it does hurt them, but they get into this restless state when they will not keep still.

When the patients are restless, find out whether it eases them or not. If it does not, they are probably Bryonia cases. If it does ease them, consider one of the other drugs—possibly Baptisia or one of the restless drugs, such as Rhus tox. It is a point that needs early clarification.

Bryonia patients feel hot, and are uncomfortable in a hot stuffy atmosphere; they like cool air about them. This can be linked with their thirst. They are always thirsty, and their desire is for cold drinks—large quantities of cold water—though, as mentioned above, they may ask for cold, sour things and then refuse them when they are brought. . . .

All Bryonia influenzas have very intense headaches. Usually, the headache is intense, congestive and throbbing; the most common situation for it is in the forehead.

Patients often say they feel as if they have a lump in their foreheads, which is settling right down over their eyes. The pain modality of the headache is that it is very much relieved by pressure—firm pressure against the painful forehead affords great relief to the Bryonia headache.

As one would expect, the headache is very much worse from any exertion—talking, stooping or movement of any kind. It is worse if the patient is lying with the head low; the most comfortable position is semi-sitting up in bed, just half propped up. . . .

As a rule, Bryonia patients do not have a very profuse nasal discharge. More commonly, they complain of feelings of intense burning and heat in the nose, or of fullness and congestion.

EUPATORIUM PERFOLIATUM (Thoroughwort)

The outstanding point which leads to the consideration of Eupatorium is the degree of pain which the patients have.

There are very intense pains all over—of an aching character —which seem to involve all the bones of the skeleton, arms, legs, shoulders, back, hips, and, particularly, the shin bones.

As a rule, Eupatorium influenzas develop rather more quickly than others, and the pains develop very rapidly. The patients say it feels as if the various joints were being dislocated—it is that type of very intense, deep-seated pain. Associated with the pain, there is incessant restlessness; the patients are always moving to try to ease the aching pain in one or other of their bones.

In Eupatorium influenzas—a useful differentiation point— the sweat is very scanty. Other drugs which have a very similar degree of bone aching all tend to sweat.

The patients are always depressed, but with a different depression from that of Bryonia. They are acutely depressed and definitely complaining; they complain bitterly about the intensity of their pain and, if they are not complaining, they move around in bed, groaning and moaning; and are very sorry for themselves.

In appearance, they usually have a fairly bright flush and a dryish skin, with rather pale lips, in contrast to the deep congested appearance in the other drugs already described. They tend to have a white-coated, thickish fur on the tongue and, instead of the bitter taste of Bryonia, they simply have a flat, insipid taste.

Eupatorium patients are always chilly; they feel cold and shivery, are sensitive to any draught of air and very often have a sensation of chilliness spreading up the back.

They usually suffer from quite intense headaches. Typically, they complain of extreme soreness of the head, very often most marked in the part that is resting against the pillow....

RHUS TOXICODENDRON (Poison Oak)

The onset of a Rhus tox. influenza is usually gradual and without a very high temperature; it is a slowly progressing feverish attack, which is accompanied by very violent generalised aching.

The aching in Rhus tox. is very typical indeed. The patients are extremely restless; their only relief lies in constant movement, constant change of position. If they lie still for any length of time, their muscles feel stiff and painful, and they turn and wriggle about in search of ease. This constant restlessness is the most noticeable thing about Rhus tox. patients on first sight.

They are very chilly, and very sensitive to cold. Any draught or cold air will aggravate all their conditions, and is enough to aggravate their coryza and start them sneezing; an arm outside the bedcovers becomes painful and begins to ache, and so on.

Understandably, Rhus tox. patients are extremely anxious; they get no peace at all, and are mentally worried, apprehensive and extremely depressed. The depression is not unlike that of Pulsatilla; the patients go to pieces and weep.

With all the restlessness and worry, they become very exhausted and, considering that their temperature is quite moderate, unduly tired-out, almost prostrated.

Rhus tox. patients invariably have extremely bad nights. It is very difficult for them to get to sleep because of their constant discomfort; when they do sleep, their sleep is very disturbed, full of all sorts of laborious dreams—either that they are back at work, or making immense physical effort to achieve something.

They sweat profusely. And the sweat has a peculiar sourish odour, the sort of odour one used to associate with a typical case of acute rheumatic fever.

These patients always have intensely dry mouths and lips, and very early in their disease they develop a herpetic eruption which starts on the lower lip—small crops of intensely sensitive vesicles that spread to the corners of the mouth. These usually develop within the first twelve hours of their illness. . . .

Rhus tox. patients have very violent attacks of sneezing. They describe them as usually more troublesome at night, and so violent as to make them ache from head to foot. As a rule, the nasal discharge is somewhat greenish in colour. . . .

They suffer from rather severe occipital headaches, with a sensation of stiffness down the back of the neck and, very often, marked giddiness on sitting up or moving. They often complain of a sensation of weight in the head, as if it were an effort to hold it up.

Rhus tox. patients often complain of a feeling of intense heat inside, and yet their skin surface feels the cold. They are sweating profusely and any draught seems to chill them— they feel the cold on the surface—but they feel burning inside.

These are only highlights of four remedies commonly used in influenza, but they should be enough to show the wide variety of symptom complexes which can occur with even such a straightforward ailment as influenza. Homeopathic prescribing is a detailed and complex affair requiring astute self-observation and reporting by the patient, and thorough skill and knowledge by the prescriber.

IX

The Patient's Responsibility

The homeopathic practitioner is faced with a challenging task in choosing precisely the correct remedy at each stage in a patient's treatment, but the patient as well carries significant responsibilities. Homeopathy is a powerful and effective therapy, but it also demands a great deal of the patient. One doesn't get something for nothing. The patient must learn to observe areas of life which are ordinarily ignored by most people, and this observation must be done objectively and dispassionately.

It is not enough for the patient to merely keep a notebook of every detail and then leave it to the prescriber to decide which details are significant and which are not. Symptoms are manifestations of the vital force, and as such they are the basis for making a homeopathic prescription. The symptoms important to the homeopath are those which have meaning to the patient, not mere pieces of data reported out of a compulsion to be "complete." Those observations noted by the patient in the course of daily existence—those which have some meaning, however small—are the very symptoms which are created by the organism's vital force, and therefore these are the ones which lead to a prescription.

On the other hand, it is important that the patient not go too far in the other direction either. Some people are too careful about not misleading the prescriber, and so they ignore changes until they are absolutely certain. For example, if a patient of this type notices a definite tendency to chilliness on a particular afternoon, his mind may search for possible explanations—perhaps someone turned down the heat, or perhaps he drank a little too much ice water at lunch, or perhaps his metabolism is lower than normal because his sleep was restless the night before. If one searches hard enough, it is possible to "explain away" virtually everything. This approach can present a big problem for the homeopath because there will be too few symptoms upon which to prescribe.

So, it is possible to go too far in either direction—either reporting too many symptoms having little actual significance, or "explaining away" the many symptoms which in fact are important. The best policy lies in between. The patient should accept the fact that everyone is an individual, including especially himself, and that any eccentricities which occur are simply a manifestation of his individuality. At the same time, the patient should not place *ultimate* importance on these changes; he should refrain from interpreting what he observes. Otherwise, he may begin to imagine that he has some serious disease, or that he is sicker than he really is. This is why I recommend an objective and dispassionate attitude. Symptom observations are just that and no more; they are observations. No judgments are made about them. They are merely manifestations of the unique way that the defense mechanism is attempting to maintain balance.

The basic task of the patient is to report to the prescriber every deviation from natural function, not only on the physical level, but on mental and emotional levels as well. Homeopaths do not limit themselves to merely physical symptoms leading to an allopathic diagnosis. Much more important are the wide variety of symptoms expressing themselves in every aspect of the patient's life—relationships, work stresses, reactions to environmental changes, food cravings or aversions, sexual desire, quality of sleep, etc.

Even small observations which seem insignificant from an allopathic standpoint may well be crucial from the homeopathic perspective—particularly if it is something which has meaning to the patient. For example, suppose a patient has been found by allopathic doctors to be suffering from ulcerative colitis. He is used to spending the entire consultation discussing details about his bowel habits. A homeopath is also interested in this information to some extent, of course, but much more time will be spent on other aspects of the patient's life. To the homeopath, the most useful information might be that the patient is often anxious—particularly about the future—is easily startled by sudden noises, can fall asleep only while lying on the right side, and has a strong craving for salt. Such pieces of information are irrelevant in the allopathic context, but they lead directly to the curative medicine in the homeopathic setting.

Another responsibility of the patient is to avoid impatience. This is especially true for chronic disease sufferers. One cannot expect immediate relief from symptoms possibly caused by pain-killers, tranquilizers, or cortisone. Homeopathy does not have specific medicines to relieve pain, allay anxiety, counteract insomnia, etc. Homeopathic prescriptions are always designed to bring about cure of the entire organism. The goal is harmonious functioning on all levels of being, not merely momentary relief of specific symptoms. Sometimes this process takes weeks or months, and in more severe cases it can take one or two years.

One must not be too impatient. Patients sometimes consult homeopaths with the idea that a miracle is likely to occur, and when progress is slower than they expect, they denounce homeopathy and seek another therapy. The laws of Nature proceed at their own pace, and they do not progress any faster under the demands of impatience.

The actual time required for cure depends upon several factors. The first is the strength of the vital force at the outset of treatment. A patient with a strong constitution will respond more dramatically, while someone with a weak vitality will take longer to cure. Stronger patients may need only one prescription, and weaker ones may need a carefully-prescribed series of remedies.

The strength of the defense mechanism is determined to a large extent by hereditary factors. Patients coming from families exhibiting many chronic diseases are likely to require a longer time for cure. In addition, patients with a history of severe illnesses, particularly if treated with many allopathic drugs, present more problems for homeopathic treatment. And finally, patients with long histories of poor diet, no exercise, and abuse of alcohol or drugs can expect cure only after extended periods of time.

Another factor in homeopathic treatment is the length of time the homeopath takes to find the indicated remedy. This is not an easy task and it may take some time to accomplish. Patients who are used to the allopathic method of prescribing, which requires relatively simple judgments for finding palliative medications, may be disappointed at first with the systematic, painstaking process involved in homeopathic prescribing. Rarely, homeopaths encounter patients who become suspicious about the competence of the prescriber when he spends so much time consulting his books and carefully inquiring into seemingly irrelevant details. The patient, however, must remember that the process of finding a correct remedy is difficult enough without having to contend with a suspicious or impatient patient. Therefore, the patient should be glad to see the homeopath taking so much time and care. The patient should try to help the homeopath feel as psychologically at ease as possible in order to aid the process.

Another factor governing the length of time for cure is the level upon which the predominance of symptoms reside. Patients suffering primarily physical symptoms are generally easier to treat than patients suffering mostly from mental or emotional complaints. This is because the vital force, insofar as possible, always tries to limit disturbances to the most peripheral levels of the organism. People can suffer from physical difficulties and still maintain a considerable degree of well-being on mental or emotional levels, but the reverse is not true. People who are disturbed on these deep levels experience much less well-being and are generally much more limited in their life-expressions. For this reason, patients with primarily mental or emotional problems have relatively weak vital force, and cure can be expected to be correspondingly slower.

Once a prescription has been made and progress has occurred, the patient still has responsibilities. There are a number of influences which can interfere with the action of homeopathic remedies. In the absence of these factors, remedies may literally continue to act for months or even years; but if the effect is disrupted, it makes further prescribing even more difficult.

Allopathic drugs are one of the most powerful interfering factors. An occasional aspirin for temporary aches or pains is generally no problem, but consistent use of analgesics, tranquilizers, antibiotics, contraceptive pills, and especially cortisone can completely counteract the action of homeopathic remedies. In some instances, even dental work can produce the same effect. Therefore, homeopathic patients should refrain from all other therapies except for true emergencies and, if possible, only after consulting the homeopath first.

Coffee is another common homeopathic "antidote." Coffee is a stimulant which can have effects as powerful as medicines. Individual sensitivities vary widely, so that for some patients a rare cup of mild coffee may have no effect, while for others even this exposure is enough to interfere. For this reason all homeopathic patients should avoid coffee altogether. Decaffeinated coffee, black tea, and grain-based coffee substitutes are all acceptable.

The handling of remedies themselves can also be an important factor for patients taking daily doses. Even in their glass vials or paper envelopes, remedies can be destroyed by exposure to direct sunlight, strong odors (particularly the odor of camphor and other aromatic substances), and excessive heat or cold. Remedies should be stored in a shaded place of moderate temperature free of strong odors.

Finally, the responsibility which occasionally can be the most demanding for the patient is that of waiting out whatever healing crisis occurs. In the process of cure, the strengthening of the vital force may result in a temporary increase of symptoms. Usually this lasts from only a few hours to a few days, but in some cases it may take longer. If the patient doesn't understand this possibility, it may at first seem as if the homeopathic medicine is having an adverse effect, and there may be a tendency to seek allopathic relief from the exacerbated symptoms. The same confusion may occur if the patient expects to never have a relapse, when in fact his or her particular case is expected to require several remedies in order to accomplish full cure. The patient must be able to recognize what is happening and trust the judgment of the homeopath. The patient must avoid panic and await further developments.

Homeopathy is a demanding system not only for the prescriber but for the patient as well. It is not a therapy in which the patient unthinkingly reports the diagnosis of allopathic physicians, receives a pill, and is then cured. It requires a good deal of objective self-observation, an attitude of sympathy and assistance for the task confronting the prescriber, a willingness to avoid interfering factors, and the wisdom to be patient during whatever healing crises occur. For most people, these responsibilities are quite easy to meet, and the results are correspondingly gratifying.

X

Does Homeopathy Work?

When a homeopath has loved and deeply studied his work for many years, it sometimes happens that he may know the right remedy for the patient immediately. This is often wrongly called intuition. Perhaps intuition comes into it, but it is really a long, most serious acquaintance with homeopathy that makes this possible. An accomplished homeopath, Dr. Karl Konig, says:

We all know the experience, that sometimes, when seeing a patient, suddenly we are struck by the image of Drosera or Antimony. We are convinced that this is the right drug and that it will fit the patient as a key fits into its lock. How does this come about? It is not a matter of combined thought and impressions of outer symptoms, it is a sudden and immediate knowledge.[13]

In homeopathy, diagnosis is nothing more than the recognition of the drug which can cause—and therefore

[13] Karl Konig, M.D., in Brian Inglis, *Fringe Medicine* (London: Faber and Faber, 1964), p. 89.

will cure—a certain totality of symptoms. That is why homeopaths all over the world talk about their patients as being a "Sulphur case" or a "Pulsatilla case" and so on, and not a diabetes or arthritis case. They call the patient and the totality of his symptoms by the name of the remedy indicated.

These images are drawn from ordinary human experience, plus a great deal more. In Appendix I, a few characteristic remedy images are presented in order to give you an idea of the detail involved; actually, even these descriptions are only a summary, since the full description of even one common remedy would occupy 50 pages or more. Here, I will present just a few thumbnail sketches.

Undoubtedly you know some hard-driving individual, constantly working to force the world to go his way, who is often nervous and irritable, snaps at every detail, yanks the door handle off the closet if it sticks a little, comes home and takes out his work frustrations on his wife and kids. He lies awake thinking about work problems only to finally relax and fall asleep just as he must get up to go to work again. In his ailments, this person will show all the characteristic physical symptoms of Nux vomica (a Brazilian nut), and will respond dramatically physically, emotionally, and mentally to its administration—often for many months or even years without the necessity of repeating it.

Or perhaps you know a very feminine, rather plump woman, very changeable in her moods, one minute in tears, laughing the next—and all at the merest change of scenery or company—who enjoys people and talking to people (particularly about her complaint), who is socially rather passive and not likely to be a leader, yet who can suddenly be spiteful and snappish if spoken to, intolerant to heat while running about in cold weather with the skimpiest of clothing, who feels best when taking a walk in open air and worse when cooped up in a stuffy room. This woman will show a dramatic response to Pulsatilla (the Wind Flower) no matter what her physical complaints may be (a skin eruption, disordered menstrual cycle, sterility, diabetes, asthma, etc.).

Homeopathy lists in its *Materia Medica* (the formal compilation of guiding symptoms of medicines) literally thousands of substances. Their provings cover most of the symptoms which the homeopath encounters in his medical life. Naturally one can, and will, add to these resources. There is need for new research, and new provings of substances not yet fully proved.

The great advantage of homeopathic diagnosis is that it concerns itself exclusively with the patient's symptoms, and discovers from these alone the cure. For the allopath, a pathological state requiring treatment exists only when he can observe some pathological tissue change in the body— a duodenal ulcer, say, or a tumor somewhere—but for the homeopath the disturbance starts with the patient's own symptoms, which are at the same time the indication to the remedy that will cure him. To a homeopath, the patient is ill when and because he feels ill, and the malady is already far advanced when it qualifies for allopathic recognition. For the allopath, the patient is ill only if his doctor can see it in the laboratory tests. The point is that the patient is right; those very disturbances which are in the beginning his symptoms can, and ultimately do, result in the tissue changes recognized by allopathy. The homeopath comes on the scene at the beginning and may cure the functional disorders, thereby aborting the possibility of subsequent pathological tissue change. It follows from all this that if the patient has to wait for an allopathic diagnosis before he can be cured, he pays for it dearly. This is why it has been repeatedly stressed that homeopathy is the best preventive method one can follow.

In Aphorism 7 Hahnemann states it very aptly:

Symptoms alone must constitute the medium through which the disease demands and points out its curative agent. Hence the totality of these symptoms, this outwardly reflected image of the inner nature of disease, must be the chief, or only means of determining the selection of the appropriate remedial agent.

One hundred fifty years later, the late Sir John Weir, a renowned homeopath and personal physician to Queen Elizabeth of England, gave a lecture on homeopathy to the Royal Society of Medicine at which he remarked:

In conclusion let me say, that the foregoing may sound to you plausible—or the reverse. But, as practical medical men, your feeling must be, "Does it work?"

In order to show you that it does work, I will take a few of the simplest cases, exemplifying Homeopathy in some of its phases. I am not going to weary you with details, but merely relate salient points.

An officer invalided home with Trench Fever. He had been ill for a year. This man had frightful irritability of temper. His fever started always at 9 a.m. He had the usual pain, restlessness, and jerking of extremities: these worse at night. One remedy only, *Chamomilla*, has just this symptom complex: and a single dose of *Chamomilla*, in high potency, quickly cured him, and sent him back to the line.

A mother of small children, with acute food-poisoning had been vomiting and purging all night, and was supported down to our out-patient department by her husband, at 2:30 p.m., cold, collapsed, anxious—almost "done." Her symptoms were typically those of Arsenic, and *Arsenicum*, in high potency, sent her home, a couple of hours later, warm and smiling, and again, well.

You see here the rapid homeopathic action in very acute sickness. The more acute the sickness, the quicker and more complete the curative reaction.

I was asked one night, at midnight, to see a man who had had champagne and oysters for dinner, and who was doubled up with colicky abdominal pain. There were beads of sweat on his forehead. His only relief was by pressing his hands deeply into his abdomen. He could only answer in a whisper. He felt so ill that he thought there was no chance of work next day. Giving him a dose of *Colocynth* [cucumber], in potency, I timed him, and in three minutes he gave a sigh, and stretched out his legs and said, "I'm better." And he went to business next day. Here the remedy had to be *Colocynth*, not *Arsenicum*; because *Colocynth* is the only remedy with abdominal pains relieved by doubling up and pressure.

At 10:30 p.m. one night, I was called to a man suffering from urticaria—anaphylactic—after anti-tetanus serum. He was almost beside himself with fear and anxiety: very restless, couldn't keep still: certain he was going to die. Thirsty, felt hot, great fear of being alone. Very apprehensive. Everything had to be done at once. Here *Aconite* [monkshood], in the 30th potency, gave almost instant relief, and in fifteen minutes the patient was quite himself again. This was one of the most dramatic things I have ever seen.

I was once urgently called to see a patient acutely ill with rheumatic fever, who was the despair of all who came in contact with him. Nurse after nurse had had to go, and the doctor in attendance was at his wit's end. Rheumatic pains intolerable: said they were driving him crazy. A dose of *Chamomilla* brought almost instant peace: the temperature promptly dropped, and the patient got well.

One might multiply such cases indefinitely: and remember, they are common, not to any one prescriber, but to Homeopathy.

In these days of advancing science, when the foolishness of Homeopathy is proving wisdom . . . and the amazing prescience of Hahnemann is obtaining every day new confirmation, what is there to prevent the most sceptical from, at least, experimenting with the power that has come to us.

Those who test Homeopathy and make the experiment, do not escape. Over and over again doctors have studied Homeopathy, or have been commissioned to look into it, in order to expose it—only to become its most enthusiastic adherents and exponents.

I suppose not one of us has approached Homeopathy otherwise than with doubt and mistrust: but facts have been too strong for scepticism.[14]

Here are additional cases gathered at random from the literature of homeopathy, to give the reader some idea of the cures it brings about. No attempt here is made to give the exhaustive detail needed to arrive at each prescription: this would require prohibitive space. None include complete detail, some present a fair amount of detail, and most are mere summaries. Nevertheless, they should serve to demonstrate the kinds of cures produced by good homeopathy.

The cases listed here cover the sublime to the ridiculous; by and large, they are serious cases, but in actual fact, experienced homeopaths routinely see cases so difficult as to have been abandoned by allopathic medicine.

EPILEPSY[15]

Ask any neurologist what the chances of curing epilepsy, especially if caused by a head injury, might be without medication. Nil! But just observe:

[14] Sir John Weir, K.C.V.O.M.B., *Homeopathy: An Explanation of Its Principles* (London: British Homeopathic Association, 1932), pp. 20–22.
[15] Actually, in homeopathy, the name of the condition takes the name of the remedy, in this case *Calcera Ostearum*.

A young lady, eighteen years old, of fine physique, seen 20th May 1909, had been suffering from very frequent (sometimes daily) epileptic fits, with biting of tongue and frothing of the mouth, since December, 1908.

There was no apparent cause except that the girl had fallen from a swing on her head, two and a half years previously, and all treatment having proved unavailing, the medical attendant and the consultant gave it as their opinion that trephining the skull appeared to be the only course to pursue to obtain cure. Naturally, the parents, having heard of some of the good results of Homeopathy, decided to give it a trial before resorting to surgical proceedings.

After full examination of patient, jotting down the symptoms and modalities, and working them out with Kent's Repertory, *Calcarea Ostearum* [carbonate of lime], was found indicated. Calc-os. 200 was given in a daily dose for three days.

For some days afterwards the fits were much more severe and frequent, but no other drug was given, and in less than a month she had her last fit, and was restored to health. She has remained free from convulsions up to the present day (which is 6 years already, 1909–1915).[16]

PEPTIC ULCER

Nowadays, peptic ulcer is a very common problem. Allopathic treatment usually focuses on antacid therapy, requiring a constant regimen of bland diet and pills. Reduction of work stress is often recommended but rarely followed. If the case is persistent, surgery is attempted and usually results in only temporary relief of symptoms.

K.M., male, age 30.
First seen: 12/19/74
Complains about repeated gastric hemorrhage.

[16] David Ridpath, M.D., *The Homeopathician*, Vol. VI, No. 2, 1916, p. 156.

History:

Since early childhood pain in stomach and water brash.

10 years old: duodenal ulcer was confirmed by X-rays.

Crises of pains on and off, cannot remember details.

First bleeding from stomach 17 years old.

Since then 9 gastrorrhagias [bleeding from stomach].

1970, vagotomy, enteroanastomosis [ulcer surgeries].

8 months later again profuse bleeding that continued appearing about once a year. Last one a month ago.

Since, nearly every day vomiting coffee-ground-colored mucous.

Family History:

Father died from bleeding of esophagus, had varicose veins, the existence of which he ignored.

Mother had duodenal ulcer for years, extreme obesity.

Symptomatology:

Heaviness in stomach 4–5 hrs. after eating, followed by regurgitating of coffee-ground-colored liquids and some remnants of food.

Typanitic distension with rumbling and pain in hypogastrium extending to lumbar region, better curling up and pressing, better flatus. This pain in the lumbar region, sometimes severe, is better by pressing and bending backwards, which brings profuse salivation.

Pain in stomach before a meal, preventing him from eating.

Distension in abdomen and pain in lumbar region when cold is felt in abdomen.

Generals and food desires and aversions:

Worse cold, worse wet weather.

Desires: mutton, sweets, cheese, sour things.

Aversions: milk, oysters, vegetables.

Salt normal. Thirstless.

He is an unhappy fellow, having been ill all his life and not able to study or do what he likes.

Irritable.

Easily tired.

Sleep good and long, prefers lying on the left.

He was given *Millefolium* [yarrow] 200, one dose.

Two months later he is much better.

Feels calmer.

Pain in abdomen gone.

Pain in lumbar region gone.

No flatus.

Sensitivity to cold gone.

Has gained 3 kgs. in weight.

Five months later: slight stomach complaints after being in a very wet place.

Started drinking milk.

Eleven months later: he is without medicine for many months.

2 or 3 times water brash without coffee-ground-colored remnants.

He gained another 2 kgs. in weight.

He keeps no diet.

He is not sensitive to cold any more.

Until recently, when seen accompanying his mother, was well.

The frequency of hemorrhages and the absence of pain during hemorrhage, tympanitic distension, ill humor and irritability (Clarke) were the clues that guided to *Millefolium*.[17]

ALLERGIES

Allergies are rapidly becoming an increasing problem in our modern societies, partly because of the increased exposures to unnatural chemicals which may help catalyze reactions to other substances, but also because the general constitutions of all members of our societies have been declining. Again, the allopathic solution is to merely suppress the symptoms by various measures.

---

[17] I. Bachas, M.D., and G. Vithoulkas, M.I.H., *Homeotherapy* 2: 6 (Aug. 1976).

K.E., female, age 68.
First seen: 6/10/75
Complains of allergic coryza and pains in spine.

History:
1920, malaria, many quinine injections.
1926, TB
1940–44, eczema on hands and feet from autoblood vaccination.
1948, allergic coryza starts, with violent sneezing.
1968, operated for nodules left by quinine injections that formed abscesses.
After this opertion coryza and sneezing subsided.
Last year it started again.

Symptomatology:
Violent sneezing followed by running watery discharge. May last from two hrs. to two days.
Worse slight draft, though she tolerates cold open air.
Better lying warm in bed, with nose covered.
To prevent prolongation of crisis she has to lie down or sit half-lying, *motionless*, for some time. If crisis becomes severe, nose swells and she cannot breathe through it or touch it.
Since 25 years she suffers from pains in lumbar region extending down to left leg, recently also to right leg. Pain recently is worse in calves and ankles, constricting.
Cramps in left calf morning on stretching.

Generals:
Bears heat and cold the same.
Worse sun.
Wakes frequently in the night, sometimes sleepless all night.

Mentals:
Anxiety, heaviness and constricted feeling in chest, bad mood, sadness. It comes like a crisis and goes by itself.
Irritable, if irritated remains silent.

In a hurry.
Nervous trembling, better by hand work.

Food desires and aversions:
Desires: meat, fish, fat, lemon.
Aversions: salty things, almond juice, slimy food.
No thirst.

Asparagus 200 was given once and repeated after 3 months because of a relapse. There was an amelioration not only in her allergic symptoms but also in the anxiety state as well, and in her spine symptoms.[18]

GASTRITIS

Again, a situation similar to that for peptic ulcer, but generally less severe. The psychosomatic correlation is well-known to modern allopathic medicine, but this knowledge does not lead to curative treatment.

C.M., female, age 22.
First seen: 6/6/75
Complains of gastritis since 3 years.

Symptomatology:
Pains in stomach in the morning until 9 a.m.
Worse after grief.
Headaches *after vexation.*
Involuntary movements of eyelids.
Counts whatever is around her when she has to wait.
Sometimes she had delusions of lights or of colors or of voices. She feels they are unreal.
Avoids being alone in the dark.
Irritable. Worse noise, talking, worse before menses, prefers being alone with somebody around.

[18] I. Bachas, M.D., and G. Vithoulkas, M.I.H., *Homeotherapy* 2: 8 (Aug. 1976).

Feels suppressed by her mother, continuous conflict that results in revolts and going away from home.

Faints at the sight of blood.

Fear of heights.

Sensitive to music and better from it.

In a hurry, impatient.

Worse after long sleep, although she finds refuge in it to avoid conflict with family.

Prophetic dreams.

Craving for the smell of naphthalene, she gets a voluptuous feeling from smelling it.

Worse cold, cold extremities.

Late menses, better when calm.

Irritability before menses.

Desires: Farinaceous foods, *soups, vegetables.*

Thirsty for small quantities.

Aversions to *slimy* food, to milk.

The symptoms fit neither Calcarea carbonica nor Arsenicum album, but the desire for liquid food was striking, which fits *Calcarea arsenicosa* [arsinate of lime].

It was given. After a severe aggravation of headaches, which was her main complaint at the time of consultation, she got well in regard to her stomach symptoms, her headaches, and much better in her psychological state. Involuntary movements of eyelids stopped, and last—and most interesting—the craving for the smell of naphthalene disappeared.[19]

DIABETES MELLITUS

Diabetes is another disease which needs no introduction to non-medical people. Although not immediately fatal as are some diseases, diabetes is a deep and debilitating illness affecting nearly all organs of the body. Modern medi-

[19] I. Bachas, M.D., and G. Vithoulkas, M.I.H., *Homeotherapy* 2: 9 (Aug. 1976).

cine is able only to "manage" it, certainly far from being able to cure it, as every physician will readily admit.

July 2nd, 1890. Male, tall, well-formed, aged forty-seven. This illness has been coming on about three years; has lost thirty-five pounds in weight and is losing steadily. Ability to exercise steadily growing less. Sleepless nights. Two years ago had occasional attacks of diarrhoea, accompanied with abdominal suffering; after these attacks the sleeplessness increased. Sometimes the pain in abdomen keeps him awake nights. Dull aching diffused through abdomen; worse nights; worse when lying down during day. Copious perspiration on slight exertion. Very nervous, must keep in motion. Stool light colored. Violent pulsation felt in body. Strong action of the heart and full rapid pulse, 95 to 100. Had "grippe" last winter and has been losing much faster since. Greasy cuticle on the urine.

Brickdust in urine, not always. Excitement often brings on a sensation as though the head or skull is divided above the ears, and lifted up and down. Can sleep in one position as well as in another. Heat overcomes him quickly but he is not sensitive to cold. Weak from exertion of body and mind. Must arise in the night to pass urine. Quantity of urine four or five pints. Specific gravity of the urine, 1030 to 1035. Fermentation test gives sugar twelve to fifteen grains per ounce. Rumbling in abdomen. This patient has visited several allopathic physicians who had given him many strong drugs, especially *Podo.*, *Strych.* He had not received any homeopathic advice. Thirst for cold water. Smarting of anus. He has been told he had fissure of anus. A few days later after a careful study of all remedies related to the case he received *Phos.* [the element phosphorus] *cm.*, which was followed by a sharp aggravation of all symptoms.

He improved steadily without further medicine until October 31st, when his symptoms began to return. The sugar disappeared from the urine within a month, and has not since appeared.

October 31st same year *Phos. mm.* He is in perfect health, doing active brain work, and his endurance is as great as ever.[20]

LIFELONG ERUPTION OF SCALP

Any physician in general practice must be a good dermatologist. Many skin eruptions are not easy to place a diagnostic label upon, and are commonly considered insignificant to many people. To the patient, however, they can be extremely distracting; and to the doctor who has to treat such ailments without real principles to guide treatment, it can be a frustrating process.

A single gentleman, 35 years of age, came to consult me at the end of August, 1887, for a coppery eruption of his scalp that he had had so long as he could remember. Besides this eruption he complained much of chronic insomnia and failing memory. I first gave him the strong tincture of *Fagus cup.,* five drops in water night and morning, but after a month— viz, on September 30—he complained that he was no better in any respect—sleepless, forgetful, restless: the eruption bad; his breath very foul; liver slightly enlarged; spleen large and very hard.

Syph. CC. November 11, "I have slept famously"; and both he and I were of the opinion that his hair had gone darker. The eruption distinctly better.

Spiritus glandium guercus O, five drops in water night and morning.

December 12. Eruption nearly gone; the spleen pains a little now; insomnia quite a thing of the past.

Tc. Carduus Marioe. He reported himself quite well of his coppery eruption on January 13, 1888, and two years later it still continued well, and since then I have no further tidings of him.[21]

[20] J. T. Kent, M.D., *Lesser Writings,* p. 428.
[21] R. S. Hayes, *Homeopathy,* Vol. V, No. 6, 1936, p. 201.

PARALYSIS

When something goes wrong in the nervous system, modern doctors still tend to throw up their hands in despair. The nervous system is such a mystery that, even if a diagnosis can be made (which is not very often), it is extremely unlikely a therapy has been found for it. Processes in the nervous system are often inexorable and usually considered irreversible, so that the true tragedy of such a situation is a kind of living death. This tragedy is compounded many-fold when it strikes a young child.

Lad, age 6. Paralysis of left arm, oesophagus, and pharynx. Difficulty in swallowing. Liquids come out of nose. Solids cause much choking. Nasal voice. Limited motion in left arm. Cannot grasp with the hand. Pale sickly face, waxy and shiny. When talking he throws the head back. Choking when eating. Bowels constipated, no action. Ineffectual frequent urging. Trouble progressing rapidly. The attack began only a few weeks ago. No history of any kind discovered in the family. Family supposed to be psoric. Lad was poisoned by *Rhus* three years ago, self-cured. Talks and cries out when sleeping. Cannot abduct the arm, but can flex it feebly. The paralysis of left is almost complete and the right is showing signs of weakness in abduction. Rash comes out on the body in heated air. *Plumb.* [lead] *42m.* Cured in six months.[22]

CHAINS OF GLANDS, WITH EXOPHTHALMOS

The following is a case of a type common to homeopathic practice. Even with today's advanced technology, there are still many people who present with undiagnosable diseases. When an allopath is confronted with an ailment without a diagnosis, he resorts to desperation measures

[22] J. T. Kent, M.D., *Lesser Writings*, p. 483.

because he has no therapy without a diagnosis. Usually a blind guess is made, and a merely palliative treatment is instituted. To a homeopath such a case causes no anxiety, because the treatment is based on the symptoms alone—the person's response to the disease—and not on diagnosis.

I have kept William D., aged 14, for a *bonne bouche*. But for the evidence of previous cases you might think I was romancing, for this is one of the most dramatic cases I have ever seen.

He first came to London Homoeopathic Hospital in November 1918, sent on to me by Mr. Hey, from his surgical clinic, as inoperable. He had marked exophthalmos, with a pulse of 150. He had chains of lymphadenomatous glands over, behind and in front of right sternomastoid, largest, size of a walnut. And, a string of glands behind left sternomastoid, largest, size of a horsebean. He had bluish, indurated patches on both calves, studded with small ulcerations. Typical "Basin" [tuberculous lymph node enlargement]. His uncle had died of phthisis. He was a seven-months' child and delicate. *Tub. bov.* [a homeopathic preparation of bovine tuberculosis] *30,* one dose.

Six weeks later. Glands improving. *Tub. bov., 30,* one dose.

Another month (January, 1919). Glands improving. Still a chain in right neck. The scores on legs are all scabbed over; none open now, and legs much less blue. Pulse 108. Eyes still prominent. *Tub. bov. 30,* one dose.

He got *Tub. bov.,* same potency, in February and March, when "very little to be seen on calves; glands improved."

April. "Neck better, legs nearly well, right prominent." *Drosera* [sundew] *200,* one dose.

The effect was dramatic. A month later (May) he had started work (engineering). I found glands well, sores well, exophthalmos gone, pulse 80. No medicine.[23]

[23] Margaret Tyler, M.D., *Homeopathic Recorder,* Vol. XLV, No. 4, 1939, p. 363.

UREMIC CONVULSIONS

When kidneys fail in their function, toxins build up in the bloodstream resulting in a condition called uremia. When severe enough, this affects the brain and becomes fatal. It is an end stage condition. Nowadays, with kidney dialysis machines, it is possible to keep people alive, but not to actually correct the kidney problem itself.

A tall, dark, scrawny man of 72 had been having uremic convulsions. First a frightful convulsion without warning, then three or four others, with anticipating frequency and lessening intensity, then beginning all over again. The only thing the man himself could tell me about it was that he had terrific sharp pains shooting up the body through the sides of the head, then he lost consciousness. The convulsions began by jumping to his feet and struggling aimlessly with loud respiratory gurgling and snorting, frightful facial contortions and frothing at the mouth. Then falling to the floor with tonic spasm and episthotonos; then coma with deathly pallor, sunken, almost hippocratic features, copious warm sweat and feeble pulse. From this he would gradually revive and after one to three hours appear nearly normal until the next convulsion. The convulsions appeared during the daytime only but he kept the family in restless solicitude with his disconcerting snorings at night.

After a dose of *Arsenicum album 4m*, there were merely threatening symptoms once; the albuminuria disappeared and there has been no trouble since—six months.[24]

RHEUMATIC HEART DISEASE

Rheumatic fever is a particular type of infection that attacks the heart valves, the kidneys, and the joints. In the pre-antibiotic era it wreaked great havoc which is still felt today amongst older people. It is particularly fearsome

[24] R. S. Hayes, *Homeopathy*, Vol. V, No. 6, 1936, p. 201.

because of the rapid destructive effect it has on the tissue of vital organs.

Mar. 21, 1908. S.E., thirteen years old. Heart: rheumatic myocarditis. Apex beat too slow. Violent aortic beat. Mitral regurgitant murmur. Enlargement left side. Pain at times, Pulse 120. Strong pulsation in neck. Rheumatism in legs and knees. Began when four years old. Rheumatic fever six years ago. Pinworms. Catarrh. Thirst for cold drinks. Mouth—bad taste waking in morning. Teeth covered with blood in morning. Urine copious. Perspiration often at night. Must have much air at night. Room must be cool. Reclines on left side; with head high. Headaches in temples, over eyes, vertex. Cheeks red. *Ledum* [marsh tea] *10m.*

April 18. Appearance much improved. Improved generally; catarrh and all symptoms. Rheumatism appears and disappears in legs and arms. Pulse 88. *Ledum 10m.*

May 11. Sleeps with mouth closed now. Pimples forehead and around mouth.

June 9. Rheumatism now and then, slight. Eyes improved. Stomach, funny sensations—pain—after eats few mouthfuls. Stools three a day, beginning after breakfast. Urine frequent; must sit long for it to start. *Aur.* [gold] *10m.*

June 29. Itching in throat. Pulse 80, irregular. Heart strong pulsation.

July 13. Urine offensive odor, as of something spoiled. Less delay in starting. L. side pain at times; stomach? Heart pains. *Aur. 10m.*

Aug. 24 and Oct. 10. *Aur. 50m.*

Jan. 11. *Aur. cm.*

Mar. 29. Mitral regurgitation. Sensation as if beats 4 or 5 times, then stops. Rheumatism. Vertigo. Blood in mouth and on teeth in morning, when awakens. Throat, sensation of lump when swallowing. Bowels normal. R. leg cramps. *Aur. 10m.* Repeated May 8 when symptoms worse after taking cold.

June 30 and July 28. *Aur. 50m.*

Aug. 25 and Oct 6. *Aur. cm.*

When the remedy was repeated in May, 1909, there was cough with expectoration nearly all blood, from "taking cold." In June, the patient had been bathing three times a day in the Lake and had pain about the heart. Other times, pain in heart or rheumatic pains returned but a general improvement continued, and she became a strong, hearty, robust girl.[25]

RHEUMATOID ARTHRITIS

Another serious consequence of rheumatic fever, or of strep throat, is rheumatoid arthritis. Of the various kinds of arthritis, it is the most severely destructive. Modern medicine has many drugs which reduce the inflammation or pain, but no methods of actually stopping the process for good without further medication.

An elderly lady of 68 years, confined to her chair for two years from rheumatic stiffness of back, hips, and ankles with soreness of bone. Pains from the ovarian region down the face of the thighs. Numbness of both hips down outside of thighs to toes worse in heels and worse at night. Vertigo in morning, seeming to ascend into head, with momentary blindness. Easy sweating. Night sweats on back, upper arms and thighs worse after 11 p.m. Formerly had migraine beginning over either eye and moving to the opposite side, worse in the sun. As of cold water flowing over hips and thighs. Itching eczema on ankles. Severe constipation. Puts feet out of bed at night. Aggravation from wind, drafts, dampness, cold and exertion. Better, continued motion. She received a single dose of *Sulphur 12*, on November 1st, 1919, and is still improving. She now walks well, goes up and down stairs and out on the street.[26]

[25] J. T. Kent, M.D., *Lesser Writings*, p. 473.
[26] M. Boger, M.D., *International Hahnemannian Association: Trans. 41st Proceedings*, 1920, p. 251.

CARBUNCLE ON BACK OF NECK

Another relatively minor but extremely distressing problem seen daily in private general practice. Nowadays, of course, we have antibiotics which dispose of such problems easily from the usual point of view. However, the *susceptibility* is not treated by antibiotics. This is an example of how homeopathy treats the whole person to cure a local problem.

A lady aged about 30, suffered greatly from a carbuncle on the back of the neck. She had applied many domestic medicines and obtained no relief. The tumefaction seemed destined to suppurate. It was *mottled bluish* and the pain was *intense, knife-cutting* and *burning.* She was sick at the stomach to vomiting, and at night she was delirious. Her eyes were staring and there was some fever; the tongue was foul and the breath fetid. There was great *tension in the scalp and muscles of the face.* She begged for morphine to "stop that *burning and cutting." Tarentula cubensis* [the tarantula spider] *12x* one dose produced quiet immediately and the angry looking tumefaction failed to complete its work; it did not suppurate. The discoloration was gone in two days, and the hardness soon disappeared also. She regained her normal state very rapidly, and she said to me a short time ago that she had never had her old headache since that swelling left her, showing how deeply the medicine affected her whole system.[27]

INJURED KNEE

Another example of a common ailment affecting the entire system, prescribed for on general indications rather than specifics.

Case 1. Miss G., age 48 years, school teacher. Recurring attacks of anxiety and depression for many years which appar-

[27] J. T. Kent, M.D., *Lesser Writings*, p. 412.

ently responded reasonably well to *Sepia* [squid ink] or *Nux vomica* in the past. November 1962 injured right knee while dancing. NAD on X-ray.

Did not improve on physiotherapy. After two months still marked swelling and flexion deformity. At this time there was a recurrence of severe depression and she attempted suicide by car exhaust fumes. However, a neighbor spotted her and prevented her from taking her life. I sent her to an orthopaedic specialist privately and he examined her knee under anaesthesia, but could find no definite abnormality. When she next came to consult me she told me that she felt as if she had a steel band tied tightly above the knee joint. On further questioning she admitted that she had an almost irresistible desire to use foul language. She then was given *Anacardium* [marking nut] with almost miraculous results—her knee cleared up, her mental outlook changed, she began to take a new pride in her appearance, applied for a new post and was accepted, and now looks a different woman altogether.[28]

PNEUMONIA

Again, a common problem in general practice. This demonstrates homeopathy's value as an alternative to drugs.

Girl of 7 was admitted (to the *Royal London Homeopathic Hospital*) at noon (March 30th, 1918) with pain in left chest, and a definite pneumonic patch was found in left base. Temperature on admission was 104; pulse went from 128 to 148, and respiration rose from 58 to 76. *Bry. 200 two-hourly*, and in less than forty-eight hours after admission the temperature was subnormal—96.8, and the pain gone.[29]

---

[28] Dr. I. Mck. Burns, *British Homoeopathic Journal*, Vol. LIII, July, 1964, p. 186.
[29] "Little Cases," *Homoeopathy*, Vol. III, No. 9, 1934, p. 287.

XI

How Cure Occurs

So far, we have considered society's return to natural processes arising from the failure of modern medicine to deal effectively with chronic diseases. Step by step, we have followed Hahnemann through his life of discovery: the Law of Similars, the process of extracting the healing power from substances while eliminating toxicity, the concept of the vital force as the basis of health and disease, and the miasms as being the underlying cause of chronic diseases. We have been given a glimpse of what it is like to have a homeopathic case taken, and the miraculous results which occur after the correct remedy has been prescribed.

Homeopathy works, but we have yet an insufficient understanding of the nature of things to be able to say precisely *how* it works. In truth, the answer is academic, since the practitioner's first obligation is to cure, and our knowledge of homeopathy is adequate to do that. Nevertheless, the human mind is not content without answers. Within the framework of existing knowledge, here, briefly, is the best answer I can give.

It doesn't take much thought to see what the symptoms of a disease mean, what they show, what they say: They are the means by which nature fights to rid the organism of the disease. As Hippocrates aptly put it: "Through vomiting nausea is cured." It seems that each organism is possessed of a defense mechanism [a manifestation of the vital force acting in the disease state] which is set in operation as soon as this organism is invaded by an internal or external morbific agent. We know that all infectious diseases have an incubation period during which the patient is unaware that he is ill; actual symptoms appear only after this period of incubation, which may last hours, or days. Here is the first clue to the theory of the dynamic conception of disease.

In the phenomenon of illness, we see the appearance of certain symptoms. But what is the process of their creation —indeed, of any creation? When something is created by man, it is first conceived in his mind. That conception is the birth of the creation at a dynamic level. When a new machine is made, its inventor first conceives it and works it out in his mind.

This rule of the dynamic origin of creation holds for all creation, whether it be for the original creation of the universe, or of man, or of man's works. "As above, so beneath." Nature works this way, and disease is created this way as well. When a morbific agent comes in contact with a susceptible organism—and here we have, clearly, the positive and the negative, light and dark, male and female, yin and yang—then the disease is conceived on a dynamic level. Only later do we feel and see its results in the organism.

This dynamic disturbance which shakes the entire organism, starting from its center, first affects the electromagnetic field of the human body. Until recently, the very concept that the human organism is associated with an electromagnetic field has received scant attention, but modern research with field-measuring devices and Kirlian photography are demonstrating that there is a highly active electrodynamic field permeating every living organism. These fields can be measured in intensity, and they have been demonstrated to be very dynamic. From moment to moment, the field changes in intensity depending upon alterations in consciousness, emotional changes, ingestion of alcohol or drugs, and even the acquisition of illness.

The discovery of bio-electromagnetic fields is beginning to revolutionize biological thinking in the same way that Einstein revolutionized the concepts of Newtonian physics. In physics, Newton explained laws which govern the visible physical universe, and these laws remain as valid today as in Newton's time. However, observations of nature on atomic and sub-atomic levels required new concepts, and these have been provided by modern physics. Basically, these concepts recognize that matter and energy cannot be considered separate categories. They are interchangeable, and they interact constantly in the context of what is called a "field." The importance of this new perspective is stated best by Albert Einstein: "We may therefore regard matter as being constituted by the regions of space in which the field is extremely intense. . . . There is no place in this new kind of physics both for the field and matter, for the field is the only reality."

Electromagnetic fields are characterized by the phenomenon of vibration. As electrons race around atomic nuclei, they first move in one direction and then another, as viewed by an external observer. This oscillation back and forth occurs at a specific frequency which is determined by the type of sub-atomic particle and its level of energy. For our purposes, however, the significant point is that

everything exists in a state of vibration, and every electromagnetic field is characterized by vibration rates (or fre-
quencies) which can be measured.

The human organism is no exception. To grossly over-
simplify a highly complex situation, one can visualize an
individual human being as existing at a particular vibrational frequency which may change dynamically every
second depending upon the mental state of the person,
internal or external stresses, illness, etc. The electromagnetic field is very likely the "vital force" which Hahnemann referred to.

Once a morbific stimulus has affected the electromagnetic field of a person, things may progress in two ways.
If the person's constitutional state is quite strong and the
harmful stimulus weak, the electromagnetic field changes
vibration rate only slightly and for only a short time. The
individual is not aware that anything has happened at all.

If, however, the stimulus is powerful enough to over-
whelm the vital force, the electromagnetic field undergoes
a greater change in vibration rate, and effects are eventually felt by the individual. A defense mechanism is
called into action which may involve changes on mental,
emotional, or physical levels.

The defense mechanism of an organism is called into
play only when a stimulus is truly a threat to the existence
or well-being of the organism. It is only then that the
organism sets in motion processes which are felt by the
patient as symptoms. The symptoms of a disease are nothing but reactions trying to rid the organism of harmful
influences which are merely the material manifestations
of earlier disturbances on a dynamic electromagnetic level.

The function of homeopathy is to powerfully strengthen
the organism's natural defense mechanism by adding to

its resources and energy. It works in the same direction as the vital force and not against it. This direction, this natural intelligence of the vital defense, is precisely that set of symptoms that allopathy would so diligently suppress.

As all substances possess characteristic electromagnetic fields, the task of the homeopath is to find that substance whose "vibration rate" most closely matches that of the patient during illness. As discussed earlier, the vibration rate is manifested by the totality of symptoms—whether in a patient as manifestation of the illness, or in provings after administration of the remedy. When the vibration rates of patient and remedy are matched, a phenomenon occurs which is very well known to physicists and engineers as "resonance." Just as one tuning fork can stimulate vibration of another of identical frequency, so the remedy enhances the vibration rate of the patient's electromagnetic field. This results in an increase of the patient's electromagnetic field at precisely the frequency needed to bring about a cure.

Of course, to accomplish such benefit, the remedy chosen must be very close to the precise vibration rate of the patient. This is why it is important for patients to consult only fully qualified homeopaths—those who have undergone at least four years of training in reputable schools and who strictly follow the basic laws and principles of homeopathy. There are many homeopaths who possess only a partial knowledge and who frequently deviate drastically from basic principles. They administer homeopathically prepared medicines, but they cannot be called homeopaths. Although poor homeopathy cannot do active, direct harm in the same sense as toxic allopathic drugs, it can create great disruption in the vital force of the patient. If disorderly prescribing occurs over a long enough period of time, the case can become so disrupted that even a highly qualified homeopath will not be able to restore the patient's health.

Because of the principle of resonance (the Law of Similars), a remedy which does not cover all the patient's symptoms cannot have any effect; nor should it be supposed that two or three drugs taken together will collectively do the work that one is supposed to do. Logic may find it perfectly reasonable that if one drug can produce 80% of a patient's symptoms and another can produce the remaining 20%, both can be safely administered together, and jointly remove the disease. But it does not work that way. It is not a matter of quantity—adding up the required number of symptoms in a variety of drugs—but rather one of quality. In nature, these remedies are all dissimilar in quality—in vibrational frequency—and thus create dissonance with one another. As a crude analogy, we may enjoy two Beethoven sonatas, each in its own mood affecting us in a refined way; but if we were to mix them simultaneously, we would hear only a meaningless and painful dissonance. Every drug has its own vibrational frequency, and in order for it to work, it must be similar to the nature of the disorder and administered singly.

XII

More Laws of Cure

Any practitioner who goes into such detail and depth with each case—homeopath or otherwise—is bound to make many crucial observations about health and disease. Just so, homeopathy has discovered further laws of the manner in which cure occurs. As with those already mentioned, these are universal laws which apply in any field—acupuncture, herbal medicine, polarity massage, psychic healing, even allopathic medicine.

You will remember that a temporary aggravation of the symptoms is to be expected after the correct remedy has been taken, and before the cure is completed. This aggravation is hardly noticeable in acute disorders but quite definite in chronic disorders. It sometimes attains an intensity which one could well describe as a healing crisis. During such a crisis one may expect such things as sudden diarrhea, increased menstrual flow, excessive perspiration, profuse expectoration, excessive sleepiness and the reappearance of any suppressed skin eruption. The duration and intensity of the crisis are in direct proportion to the severity of the case. Two conditions are necessary for such a reaction: the correct remedy, and a vital force strong enough to produce a reaction. This explains why true homeopaths delight in such aggravations.

It often happens that in individuals of weak vitality, this curative crisis comes about only when the organism has been sufficiently strengthened, both by continuous and careful prescribing, and by the right kind of life.

In homeopathy, up to twenty-two different reactions have been found after the first prescription. It is not within the scope of this book to go into minute detail. It may simply be enough to say here that after the first prescription the symptoms may disappear in one of four directions. They may:

1. Go from the center to the circumference of the body.
2. Travel from above downwards.
3. Go from more vital to less vital organs.
4. Disappear in the reverse order of their onset—those that appeared first being the last to disappear.

By symptoms moving "from the center to the circumference" we mean that the brain, which is the seat of thinking and all higher functions, is at the center of man. With the organism considered as a whole, the brain is automatically recognized as its most vital part—its center. Next in importance comes the heart, the liver, lungs, kidneys, down to the muscles and skin, which constitute the circumference of the organism. These latter are man's least vital organs in that a scratch or the rupture of a blood vessel on the skin can safely be neglected, while on the brain the same thing could be fatal. We also know that if the center is disturbed, the whole organism suffers profoundly.

For example, when a mental case is treated homeopathically, in the course of treatment the mental symptoms disappear and are followed by violent symptoms in the stomach. By this phenomenon the homeopath knows that a complete cure will eventually come about, because the direction followed by the symptoms is correct: from the center to the circumference. Likewise, in the case of asthma, if a skin eruption appears during the treatment, it shows that the disease is moving towards the circumference, thus guaranteeing that the patient will finally be cured.

It takes a master homeopath to understand the symptoms of a patient, evaluate them correctly, and treat them accordingly. Unfortunately, after a favorable reaction the ignorant patient, anxious to clear up his skin condition immediately, often finds some obliging allopath to swiftly restore him to his previous condition.

One of those who have most clearly described the direction followed, if a cure is to take place, is Hippocrates himself. In the 49th of his aphorisms he writes: "In a person suffering from angina pectoris the appearance of swelling and erythema on the chest is a good sign, for it shows that the disease is moving towards the circumference."

And in section 7, aphorism 5: "In a mental disorder of a maniacal type, dysentery or anasarca is a good sign."

Again in section 6, aphorism 11: "In those suffering from depression of spirits and kidney diseases the appearance of hemorrhoids is a good sign."

Section 6, aphorism 21: "The appearance of varicose veins or hemorrhoids in those suffering from mania shows that the mania is cured."

And in aphorism 26 of the same section: "If the erysipelas moves from the outside to the inside, it is a bad sign, but if the opposite happens it is a good sign."[30]

[30] Hippocrates, *Aphorisms*; author's translation from the Greek.

In all these examples we can see how correctly this great physician understood and described the law of direction.

The direction "from above downwards" appears mainly in skin eruptions where the trouble moves from the head and the upper part of the extremities towards the fingers and nails. Likewise, if the symptoms move from the brain to the lungs, this is a movement from above downwards, and at the same time from a more vital to a less vital organ.

Finally, the symptoms disappearing "in the reverse order" to which they appeared means, for example, that if a patient suffered from chronic headaches ten years ago and then from vertigo and after that from depression or epilepsy, the depression or the epilepsy would be the first to disappear; next vertigo; and, then, when this had gone, the headaches would return and finally they also would disappear. This gives an idea of what detailed and careful work is required of a homeopath in each individual case if he is to restore his patients to health. It also shows the knowledge he must have and the difficulties he encounters when, in the course of treatment, old symptoms reappear and the patient is anxious to get rid of them.

It is of the utmost importance then for the patient to thoroughly know the theory of homeopathy; otherwise he will perhaps discontinue treatment just when he is improving. It has been the source of much disappointment for me to see good work undone by ignorance and impatience.

XIII

The State of Homeopathy in the World

It is not the case that science and its institutions automatically accept truth once revealed. It is a naive and romantic notion that scientists and clinicians are rationally motivated people prepared to instantaneously discard prejudice in the face of truth. The stories of Descartes, Galileo, and many other pioneers, vilified in their times, are proof enough of this.

In the case of homeopathy, it is clear that vast changes in attitudes and procedures—even in financial structures —would have to occur for its radical principles to be adopted. Such a change would involve the entire range of institutions connected with the medical establishment— medical schools, research laboratories, pharmaceutical companies, health insurance companies, the Food and Drug Administration, etc. Such widespread political and institutional changes, if possible at all, can only occur very slowly.

Great numbers of chemists, physicians, public health officials, druggists, and others with a vested interest will instantly rally to the defense of allopathy. They will tell you that modern medicine has spectacularly raised the expectation of life throughout the world. They will not admit to having helped produce the kind of man who is really dead at thirty, though he may live to seventy. Clearly, mankind's physical and mental misery continues to increase agonizingly with the years, even if his body stays alive much longer than before. Cancer, epilepsy, heart disease, insanity, and ever new varieties of physical and mental imbalance increase inexorably.

One of the most frustrating and difficult problems in homeopathy—the one probably most responsible for the relative decline in homeopathy in the past seventy years—is an economic one. Homeopathy requires a lot of time, both with the patient and in study of the case outside of the interview period. In the past, when the society was largely rural, the physician went with horse and buggy and spent a day or an afternoon with the whole family. He had the time necessary to properly take a homeopathic case—besides being able to observe first-hand the environment of the patients. He was quite content to take his time, because his payment was in chickens, having his roof fixed in the winter, or a jacket made specially for him.

When society and medicine moved into urban locations, everything became much more complicated—the physician acquired an office, had formal appointments, a nurse, a secretary, etc. Money became the medium of exchange, and overhead became a problem. In the modern world, the cost of maintaining a medical practice is enormous for any physician, and it is no less for a homeopath. The economic realities place an incredible pressure on the homeopathic practitioner to see as many patients as possible each day.

Unfortunately, working with the laws of nature does not allow for an appointment schedule; those who stick to a rapid schedule get poor results. Those who actually take the time needed for each case must charge high fees for their interviews, and they still end up spending many hours working on cases outside of the time included in the fee.

For the patient, homeopaths' fees may seem steep at first, but in reality the savings are considerable. Ailments that are quickly cured by homeopathy could have cost many thousands of dollars to be merely palliated for years by allopathic treatment.

For this reason, the true homeopath makes only a fraction of the income of his allopathic counterpart. For a young doctor graduating from school and internship, saddled undoubtedly with large debts and perhaps a growing family, this becomes a powerful disincentive. It is unlikely that hordes of medical doctors will come flocking to homeopathy in the near future.

However, even if we somehow came across an ideal situation—a community in which homeopathy could be practiced freely without political opposition, and a physician who was interested in homeopathy and was also independently wealthy—the largest obstacle of all would still have to be confronted: the extreme time and effort required to study homeopathy adequately. Obviously, homeopathy is not the sort of profession which can be learned in a few weeks or a few months by taking a seminar. Only a four-year course of pure homeopathy in a specialized homeopathic school could adequately prepare a student to practice. We will discuss the details of such training in the next chapter.

There are very few doctors with the dedication and insight to make the required sacrifices. Any medical student intending to practice homeopathy must finish six or seven years of allopathic study before he can think of studying homeopathy, and in any case this allopathic training is of little use to him in his homeopathic practice. If, after completing seven years of medical training, he still has the energy, the courage, a willing family, and the money to persist in his endeavor, he must study homeopathy privately, or in some homeopathic clinic which may be quite far from his home. Even then, the training is inadequate, and it can only mislead such a doctor into believing his partial knowledge is all there is to know. This results in an inadequate brand of homeopathy, which ultimately seriously obstructs the cause of true homeopathy. Such is the state of homeopathy in the world today, with few exceptions.

The practical problems, however, are merely a reflection of the deeper issue of the era in which we live. Technology has led to deeply ingrained ways of thinking in all of us which emphasize materialism over subtle or dynamic realities. Truth only operates in a society in direct proportion to the maturity, the civilization, the understanding, the degree of evolution of its people. Such a society in which all things have taken their rightful place, and in which man lives in right relationship to the world about him and to himself, will naturally adopt homeopathy. But can we really expect any society to mature to this degree of goodness overnight? There is no trick, no easy pill by which the enormous forces that have led to man's present predicament can be short-circuited or counteracted.

Homeopathy, which can end so much suffering, must be deserved. Only that person with intelligent understanding and insight will choose homeopathy. To them that have will be given. It is a fact, for instance, that the family physicians of countless people have ridiculed homeopathy to them and stopped them from making their own inquiries; nay, stopped them from being really cured! Is this the fault of homeopathy or the society in which we live? At the risk of perhaps being misunderstood, I should like to say again that only those who deserve it will find and benefit from homeopathy!

Homeopathy has been in the world for more than one and a half centuries: it has withstood the relentless test of time and the vicissitudes of many attacks, because it is true. In about 1845, when the French minister F. Guizot was asked by an allopathic medical committee of France to suppress homeopathy, he replied: "If homeopathy is a chimera or a method without any value, it will disappear. But if, on the contrary, it represents a progress, it will spread whatever we do to stop it; and the Academy should desire this above all, since her mission is to stimulate scientific advances and to encourage discoveries."[31]

[31] Quoted in Brian Inglis, *Fringe Medicine* (London: Faber & Faber, Ltd., 1964).

XIV

Plans for the Future

Despite the difficulties of creating a new and revolutionary system in the world, there are actually some very exciting and important steps being taken to establish and institutionalize the highest standard of homeopathy. These efforts require the assistance of many individuals in a wide variety of ways. How can an individual contribute to the establishment of homeopathy?

The first and most important thing to do is to be treated by a good homeopath. Personal experience is the only way one can fully appreciate the benefit of homeopathy. It is not necessary to have a serious disease to be treated homeopathically; virtually everyone has some disturbance or imbalance to be corrected.

How does one find a good qualified homeopath? As a first step, the resources listed in Appendix III will help. In addition, you can seek out homeopaths who have been trained extensively by the eminent homeopaths of modern times.

The ultimate goal for the future is to establish a full-time professional school for training homeopaths. At present (December 1978), the resources are not available to directly establish such an institution. Steps toward that end have already begun, however, and there is much that can be done to further this progress.

A non-profit organization has been established to promote the various projects to spread homeopathy in the world: The International Foundation for the Promotion of Homeopathy. It is located at 76 Lee Street, Mill Valley, CA 94941. The primary need is money. Donations to the Foundation are tax-deductible. But also needed are the skills and talents of all who wish to assist homeopathy to gain its rightful place in the world. Skills, talent, and, above all, imagination are the forces which will bring the truths of homeopathy into concrete reality.

An important project now in the planning stage is the establishment of a healing center to which people of various degrees of health from all over the world can come for treatment. Such a facility will not only provide the best of homeopathic care (along with other holistic therapies when indicated), but it would also be a training facility for homeopaths who have completed the basic training. This facility will then become the nucleus eventually for the formation of the full-fledged homeopathic professional school.

Such are the plans which have already been formulated. It is impossible to predict the directions of growth for such a successful and complete system of healing. But the limits are only defined by the energy, vision, and talent of those who apply themselves to the task with love for their fellow beings.

Finally, let us describe briefly the vision of the curriculum of the homeopathic school of the future. Such a curriculum would have to be radically different from anything taught in medical schools at present, and I shall try, in very broad lines, to describe what would be necessary.

To do so we must first consider the most basic subject matter of medicine: man himself.

Until now, applied medicine has considered the human being exclusively as a physio-electrochemical organism. In theory, it might admit that there is something beyond man's material body, something called the psyche, or the mind. But what do physicians really know about these matters? In their everyday practice they are called upon to treat skin eruptions that come on after deep distress, Bell's palsy after anxiety, diabetes after disappointment, duodenal ulcers after irritability or tension, insomnia caused by ambition or fear, chorea after mortification or vexation, and so on without end. So they know in their practice the effects that disturbed thoughts and feelings have upon the body. Yet they have neither the knowledge nor the means to go to the root of these disorders, nor do they ever stop to think that some other treatment may be needed.

It is indispensable to teach the practicing homeopath about the mind and the emotional sphere of mankind. The homeopathic *Materia Medica* deals exhaustively with all these, and therefore the homeopath has the means to detect all disturbances, trace their origins, and treat them radically. Hence, homeopathic *Materia Medica* will be one of the main subjects taught throughout the entire period of study.

Next comes what is called homeopathic philosophy, which deals with the laws and principles that govern a cure. This will cover not only those considerations described in this book, but also many more which enable the homeopath to recognize quickly when a cure is in progress, when the disease is being suppressed, when to wait for further elucidation of progress, how to discover the "essence" of a given case, what cases are curable or incurable, etc.

Then the student will be taught all the subjects that will give him or her accurate knowledge of how the human body is constructed and functions in health and disease: anatomy, physiology, pathology, pharmacology, and the various specialties. These subjects, however, will be taught in a new light, always from the knowledge of the action of the vital force. In this way many things that remain mysterious to even modern medicine will be explained. The student will also be taught everything in modern technology that is relevant to the healing art—such as laboratory diagnosis, X-ray interpretation, electrocardiographic interpretation, etc.—as well as the elements of certain ancient and modern holistic techniques that have proved effective in certain instances.

Then the student will have to be taught through the living example of his teachers that love and compassion constitute the rules on which he should build his scientific knowledge, if he really wants to help his patients.

Finally, the teachings of the school should be such as to bring about, in the very depths of the students' hearts, the realization that the human being is not an accidental event, but the result of a Divine Order or Will, and that its destiny is to free itself from the bondages of pain, of passion, and of selfishness.

XV

Promise for the New Age

I strongly believe that humanity is entering a New Age in consciousness, a new understanding of things, making deep changes, re-evaluating accepted norms—in short, that there has begun a deep and sincere revolution leading to a spiritual evolution unprecedented in strength and eagerness until this time.

One catalytic factor forcing humanity to this re-evaluation is *suffering*, and a great deal of this is due to humanity's state of health.

As people awaken now to a new dimension in the understanding of existence and their relationship to the world in general, they find themselves crippled, for the tool, the means through which they may attain a higher state— namely the body—has degenerated to the point of incapacity.

The intelligent person soon asks the question, "If orthodox medicine were really good and effective, wouldn't it have improved the situation? How is it then that we see today millions of epileptics, insane, paranoids, diabetics, asthmatics, heartsufferers, and cancer victims?"

It is therefore natural that people turn to an alternative.

In this small treatise, I have tried to show the depth and thoroughness of homeopathy, and its unbelievable effectiveness. Needless to say, we need Masters in homeopathy to perform the miracle, but the main thing is that it can be done. It is not only I who make this statement, but every Master of the past and present.

The following is from a speech by Dr. W. H. Schwartz during an international homeopathic congress in America:

Let me present the evidence of my Master, James Tyler Kent, A.M., M.D., taken from his presidential address to the Society of Homeopathicians in Chicago, 1912:

"Let us announce to the world WHAT we can do, if we do it, that it may be a standard for others to follow. All acute diseases, no matter how painful and malignant they may be, may be aborted or cured by homeopathy: typhoid and whooping cough within ten days; la grippe, acute bronchitis, pneumonia, remittent fever within a few hours; scarlet fever, diphtheria, intermittent fever, measles and smallpox within a few days; septic fevers within a few hours."

I once asked Dr. Kent, "What can you do for the insane?" for I knew of some remarkable cures he had made. He replied, "I could go through our insane asylums and take out about half of them and cure them, and if I could have reached them at the time they were incarcerated, I could have cured practically all of them excepting those cases due to imbecility, tumours, and epilepsy."

All expert homeopaths will attest to Dr. Kent's announcement as being verified by their individual experiences. Your experience will prove that homeopathy is a talisman from which all diseases fade away. It is specific.

Yet in spite of claims by Hahnemann more than one hundred years ago with demonstrated proof; Dr. Kent's announcement twenty years ago; and your individual experiences, we are slow to let the world, both professional and laity, KNOW what homeopathy can do. How could they know if WE do not tell them? We tell one another often in our societies and journals, but we have neglected to "go out into the world and preach the Gospel."

We are lazy, and we alibi with "professional ethics." We follow the path of least resistance preferring to be entertained, amused and "letting George do the work." We are like the foolish virgins: we bury our talents and hide our candle under a bushel measure, keeping suffering humanity in the dark. Is that ethical? It is our duty to go out and preach, ADVERTISE homeopathy. The medical profession at large is starving and wants homeopathy but they don't know that they do. . . .

If someone had the genius to awaken the world and make it realize what homeopathy can do, it would mean a new epoch for humanity—a renaissance in medicine. Indeed, homeopathy is so far-reaching that its universal use in medicine would mean great progress toward the millenium, as homeopathy has to do with not only the physical but spiritual development in man—the homeopathic remedy actually saves souls in this way. It assists in destroying the evils by creating harmony of the physical organs and thus promoting a pure vehicle for intellect and spirit to function. Homeopathy helps to open the higher centres for spiritual and celestial influx. It is the only scientific system of medicine, but is too difficult to master without intensive training. . . .

Homeopathy is not limited to certain diseases but is universally applicable to all diseases. It cannot cure all cases as in some there is not sufficient vitality that may be aroused to cure.

There is another field of homeopathic achievement. Without fear of being challenged by the expert homeopathic physician, I will state that practically every individual may have many years added to his life if taken in time, by being vitalized by the homeopathic constitutional remedy. Even those elderly souls who ordinarily would have died at three score years and ten, in many instances, can be rejuvenated, vitalized and given a new lease of life, adding years of usefulness and comfort, and joy to their family. It was this fact that led me to prophesy in one of my writings in 1916 that Mr. John D. Rockefeller would undoubtedly live to be over 90 years of age, for I knew his physician, Dr. Alonzo Austin, had vitalized this remarkable man with homeopathic remedy.[32]

Homeopathy is absolutely effective in cases where there are no pathological tissue changes—that is, in cases where the disorder is still only functional. In such cases, though the sufferings of the patient may be intense, no seat of the disease appears, even after the most thorough clinical examinations. Homeopathy also has most spectacular results in diseases of children, both acute and chronic. In children, the disease has not had time to progress to the point of being incurable. The vitality of children is also still at its height and therefore capable of bringing about the necessary reaction. A child treated by homeopathy will grow with far less suffering than another, because homeopathy eliminates his predispositions towards disease. Of course, if predisposition to any disease is going to be completely eliminated, the treatment must be continuous and should start at the very beginning of life—conception.

Therefore, homeopathy can regenerate the population of any country that adopts it completely, together with some other auxiliary sanitary measures which are not within the scope of this book.

It often happens, if the doctor is a real master of homeopathy, that even cases considered incurable can be restored to health through continuous and proper stimulation of the vital force. That is why Dr. J. T. Kent, the man who effected the most spectacular cures in the world of homeopathy, wrote as follows to one of his friends: "My records of epilepsy, blindness, cancer, etc., I dare not publish, as I

[32] William Henry Schwartz, M.D., *Homeopathy*, Vol. V, 1936, pp. 15–18.

would certainly be hounded as a falsifier. I should not believe it myself unless I had seen the patients come and go."[33]

Homeopathic journals all over the world are full of cures in cases like asthma and all kinds of allergic conditions of the lungs and higher respiratory tract, anemias, skin afflictions of all kinds—like psoriasis and dermatitis, rheumatoid arthritis, heart disease, kidney and liver complaints, chronic headache, vertigo, mental disorders, and so on. Most of these have been declared incurable by allopathic medicine; all of them have been cured by homeopathy.

This is the main reason why homeopathy has survived and spread as widely as it has. It is at present practiced in nearly every country of the world. Now that this is so, now that it has cured millions of people, we can understand the meaning of the epitaph which Hahnemann chose for himself: *Non Inutilis Vixi*—"I did not live in vain."

It would be fitting to end this book with the words that Hahnemann bequeathed to coming generations:

"Refute these truths if you can by showing a still more efficacious, certain, and agreeable method than mine; refute them but not by words alone, for we already had too many of those. But if experience should prove to you, as it has to me, that my method is the best, make use of it to save your fellow-creatures and give the glory to God."[34]

[33] *James Tyler Kent: Physician–Teacher–Author* (Homeopathician Publishing Co., Pittsburgh, Pa.), reprinted from the *Homeopathician*, July–Sept., 1916.
[34] S. Hahnemann, *Organon of Medicine.*

Materia Medica

Following are a series of typical homeopathic remedy images. These papers are designed to convey the "essence" or "soul" of the remedies, as well as some concept of the stages of development of their pathology. These are only a few of the hundreds of remedies well-known to all competent homeopaths, and these descriptions represent only a small fraction of the wide variety of symptoms seen in each remedy. (Remember, in homeopathy the condition and the remedy take the same name.)

In reading these descriptions, do not forget that the actual prescription of a homeopathic remedy is not based upon the personality of the patient, but upon pathological states. The goal of treatment is not to alter the personality of the patient, or to get rid of healthy manifestations of the uniqueness of the individual, but rather to remove limiting factors in order to allow the individual a greater degree of freedom.

Nux Vomica (Brazilian Poison Nut)

Nux vomica is one of the more commonly prescribed remedies in the homeopathic *Materia Medica*, being one of the remedies absolutely essential for every homeopath to know in depth. To begin with, we will describe the type of person most commonly affected by Nux vomica, and then describe in more depth the peculiar Nux vomica pathology. Generally, the Nux person possesses a husky, solid, compact, muscular body type, a basically strong constitution. He is ambitious, intelligent, quick, capable, and competent. Frequently, his upbringing emphasizes a strong sense of duty, and strongly values the work ethic. The Nux person is self-reliant, rather than dependent. His intelligence is pragmatic and efficient rather than philosophical or intellectual. The Nux person, in the non-pathological state, makes an excellent, hard-working, efficient employee—and his talents lead him toward such occupations as supervisors, managers, businessmen, accountants, salesmen.

As always in homeopathy, however, we must be careful not to prescribe Nux vomica on the basis of such positive and constructive personality traits. Unlike the techniques of astrology, palmistry, handwriting analysis, physiognomy, and others which describe the qualities of a person— whether for good or bad—homeopathy bases its prescriptions on the *pathological* state of the person. We would not wish to give a remedy which might make a person less pragmatic and efficient! So, let us consider the stages in the development of the pathological state requiring Nux vomica for cure.

In the first stage, the Nux person demonstrates an exaggeration, and excess, of the normally beneficial qualities of ambition and conscientiousness. Instead of using his talents merely to work in an appropriate, relaxed, and balanced manner, the Nux person begins to become ruled by them. The ambition begins to occupy him during all the hours of the day and night, becoming a *driving* ambition, an over-emphasis on achievement and competition. Nux is the most competitive remedy in the *Materia Medica*, competitive to the point of damaging his own health and even at the expense of his colleagues. The Nux person can become a workaholic, dominated by work. Because he is capable and efficient, it is likely that he will be rapidly promoted to greater and greater responsibilities. The Nux person will welcome such promotions. Two other remedies with similar physical symptomatology, Arsenicum and Phosphorus, will take different attitudes. Arsenicum will tend to decline a promotion with too much responsibility, partially because of insecurity, partially because the self-centered Arsenicum person is more interested in personal comfort than achievement. The Phosphorus patient may be intelligent and quick also, but will shrink from the intense competitiveness which might be necessary to get ahead.

In Nux vomica, the normally conscientious state can be exaggerated out of proportion, leading to a compulsive efficiency. Nux is one of only a few remedies listed under the rubric Fastidious—but specifically the Nux fastidious-ness is tied to the emphasis on efficiency. In this sense, Nux fastidiousness is more appropriate to reality and not so severely pathological as would be assumed by its designa-tion in italics in the Repertory (a massive cross-reference to homeopathic symptoms and remedies). The Arsenicum fastidiousness, on the other hand, is a typical example of the severe, neurotic fastidiousness so classically described by psychiatrists. It is a compulsively neurotic concern with cleanliness and order both, arising out of a deep-seated anguished feeling of insecurity; the Arsenicum patient is constantly straightening and cleaning, far in excess of what is required for simple efficiency. Natrum muriaticum is an-other well-known fastidious remedy; in this case, it is more a concern with punctuality and scheduling of time, as well as cleanliness and order.

Eventually, the Nux vomica person may end up in a job which is over his head. Typically, he responds by working harder and longer, expecting more from himself and others. The Nux person characteristically carries the implicit assumption that any challenge, any problem, can be overcome by sheer effort and ability. One of the most difficult things for a Nux patient to do is to accept a limitation, or to resign himself to the inevitable. To keep up with the pressure, he comes to use various artificial means to keep himself stimulated—coffee, cigarettes, drugs (whether by prescription or social drugs such as marijuana), alcohol, and even sex. Despite such abuse of stimulants, it is also true that Nux patients are unusually sensitive to many of these substances and consequently suffer consequences of their indulgences.

The Nux vomica person is known to be a hyper-sexual individual. He has a very strong sexual desire, and may indulge his sexual impulses even beyond the bounds of conventional morality. Despite being bound by the work ethic, the Nux person is not the typical upright, moralistic personality. In his use of stimulants and drugs, and most particularly in the sexual sphere, his behavior is conducted out of impulse and therefore is best described as "amoral." As in the rest of the Nux picture, over-indulgence of sex finally results in a state of exhaustion; in later stages, the Nux patient suffers from impotence, typically a loss of erection upon intromission.

The over-indulgence of stimulants may meet his needs for awhile, but eventually the over-stimulation and toxicity take their toll. The stomach becomes disordered. The entire nervous system becomes overwhelmed and oversensitive. Even slight stresses such as light, small noises, someone's voice, or singing, become intolerable. The effects of this "over-amped" nervous system are described brilliantly by Kent: "For example, a business man has been at his desk until he is tired out, he receives many letters, he has a great many irons in the fire; he is troubled with a thousand little things; his mind is constantly hurried from one thing to another until he is tortured. It is not so much the heavy affairs but the little things. He is compelled to stimulate his memory to attend to all the details; he goes home and thinks about it; he lies awake at night; his mind is confused with the whirl of business and the affairs of the day crowd upon him; finally brain-fag comes on. When the details come to him he gets angry and wants to get away, tears things up, scolds, goes home and takes it out on his family and children. Sleeps by fits and starts, wakens at 3 a.m. and his business affairs crowd on him so that he cannot sleep again until late in the morning when he falls into a fatiguing sleep and wakens up tired and exhausted. He wants to sleep late in the morning."

The nervous system seems to become bound up, works against itself. Again, this is described best by Kent: "Another state running through Nux is that actions are turned in opposite directions. When the stomach is sick, it will empty its contents with no great effort ordinarily, but in Nux there is retching and straining as if the action were going the wrong way, as if it would force the abdomen open; a reversed action; retches, gags, and strains and after a prolonged effort he finally empties the stomach. The same condition is found in the bladder. He must strain to urinate. There is tenesmus, urging. The bladder is full and the urine dribbles away, yet when he strains it ceases to dribble. In regard to the bowels, though the patient strains much, he passes but a scanty stool. In the diarrhea at times when he sits on the commode in a perfectly passive way, there will be a little squirt of stool, and then comes on tenesmus so that he cannot stop straining, and when he does strain there comes on the sensation of forcing back; the stool seems to go back; a kind of anti-peristalsis. In constipation the more he strains the harder it is to pass a stool."

These are the patients complaining of gastritis or ulcer or "spastic colon." They finally go to the doctor, who pronounces their condition psychosomatic and prescribes ant-acids, antispasmodics, tranquilizers, or even psychotherapy. These merely mask the symptoms, usually ineffectively, and consequently worsen the sensitivity of the nervous system in general.

The Nux patient, then, is very irritable, but this is a kind of irritability which the homeopath may find difficult to elicit without care. The Nux patient will tend to hold the irritability inside (at least in this early stage). You ask, "Are you irritable?" The patient says, "No, not at all. I never even raise my voice." So you ask, "How about inside? Do you feel irritable inside yourself?" Patient: "Oh, yes! Very much!!" It is such people who are most prone to gastritis and peptic ulcer. If the person were to learn to be more expressive, he would be spared the ulcer—but then, the abuse of coffee, cigarettes, and alcohol might result in the same condition, anyway.

Finally, the pressures become too much and the Nux patient becomes impatient and irritable. He becomes impatient with himself, and particularly with others, scolding and reproaching others over minor incidents. He reacts impulsively over small disturbances. Someone quietly whistles a tune, and he yells, "Can't you keep quiet?" He can't find a pencil, so he slams the desk drawer shut. He has momentary difficulty buttoning his shirt, so he rips the button off. Someone contradicts him, and he stalks out

of the room while loudly slamming the door. He is intolerant to contradiction, but not so much from arrogance or
haughtiness (like Lycopodium or Platina), but rather because he is certain he is right and is impatient with others
who have not thought the problem through as quickly as
he; and, indeed, he *is* most often right. His impulsiveness
can lead to many personnel difficulties; Nux vomica patients are blunt and undiplomatic, and therefore would
not make very good politicians by nature.

In the next stage of development, Nux becomes actually
malicious, cruel, violent. Cruelty may begin by talking
behind the backs of others, behavior arising out of the
competitive instinct. He may, simply out of a cruel impulse, kick animals (like Medorrhinum). As this progresses,
Nux may become outright violent; most likely, many hus-
bands who beat their wives or parents who commit child
abuse would benefit from Nux (if the rest of the image
fits, of course). The violence is not necessarily focussed
always on others; Nux also can have a suicidal disposition.

The final stage of Nux is a state of insanity, a paranoid
state. The Nux patient is constantly tormented by the
impulse to kill others, but may not manifest actual violence. A woman may be haunted by a desire to throw her
baby in the fire, or to kill her husband. In the Repertory,
Nux is listed under a variety of delusions having to do
with murder, being murdered, being injured or insulted,
and of failure. To the external observer, however, the
internal torment of the Nux patient may not be at all
evident. This is the stage when Nux has an aversion to
company and refuses to answer questions. It is a state of
mental disorder which may appear very much like that
described in the last stage of Arsenicum; although a careful history of the stages of development of the pathology
will make the distinction very clear. Nux is self-reliant,

independent, compulsively hard-working, overly efficient, and irritable and impulsive; while Arsenicum is insecure, dependent, concerned about personal health and comfort, compulsive about cleanliness and order, and very anxious.

Considering the physical level of the Nux image, a general impression is that Nux vomica primarily affects functional difficulties. It does not have the deep degenerations that are characteristic, for example, in Arsenicum, which has deep spreading ulcerations and gangrenous putrefactions.

Nux vomica affects the nervous system very strongly. There are initially many twitchings and jerkings, similar to those in Hyoscyamus and Agaricus. There are severe neuralgic pains, particularly of the head. Nux is often needed in apoplectic states, especially in cases in which the paralysis is accompanied by pains in the affected limbs. In more extreme disorders, there are convulsions, opisthotonos, epilepsies. Considering the abuse of drugs like alcohol, it is not surprising that Nux vomica is a remedy which might be indicated in delirium tremens.

All beginning students of homeopathy are taught the generalities of Nux vomica: chills, worse from drafts, worse in the morning. Nux is one of the chilliest of remedies; however, it tends specifically to be more aggravated in cold, dry environments and ameliorated in wet weather (along with Asarum, Causticum, and Hepar sulphur). Nux is very sensitive to drafts, which can easily cause a coryza if the patient has perspired (which occurs easily in Nux from slight exertion). A peculiar characteristic of Nux coryzas is that the nose is stuffed up while outdoors and flows fluidly indoors; also, the nose runs freely during daytime and stuffs up at night.

The gastrointestinal tract is particularly sensitive in

Nux. As mentioned, gastritis and peptic ulcer are commonly seen, causing spasms, eructations, gagging, and retching which are unsatisfying to the patient. There is great sensitivity to almost all kinds of food; in the broken-down Nux state, especially, there will be very little appetite, and the patient will be found to be a very picky eater. There is an aversion to meat, yet there may be a desire for fat—as well as for stimulants, pungent things, and spices which are craved for their stimulating effects but which may disorder the stomach. The Nux patient will report that he becomes sick whenever his stomach is disordered; he gets a cold, a headache, or asthma. Pains in the abdomen are commonly accompanied by the desire for stool which so frustrates Nux.

As is commonly seen in alcoholics, the Nux system may commonly show congestion of the portal system—esophageal varices, and particularly hemorrhoids. There is also a tendency to jaundice, corresponding in many instances to cirrhosis of the liver. Nux will sometimes relieve the spasm of gallstone colic, enabling the stone to pass into the intestinal tract; it may also relieve renal stone colic in the same manner.

In conclusion, it is important to be reminded that the symptoms described in this paper are not designed to be exhaustive, but merely to present an image, to point to the "essence." In any given patient, any combination of such symptoms may be there, perhaps excluding some classic symptoms of Nux, and yet the patient will still require this remedy. In most cases, the obsession with tasks or work, the irritability from the overextended nervous system, and the chilliness will be there. But, for example, a particular patient may avoid alcohol and dislike cigarettes and yet still need Nux vomica. In homeopathic prescribing, we are not matching symptoms *per se*; rather, we are matching the essence of the patient with the essence of the remedy.

Lycopodium (Club Moss)

Lycopodium is one of the deepest and broadest acting medicines in the entire *Materia Medica*, potentially affecting all conditions known to mankind. Despite its wide application, however, there is a central thread which runs through the remedy and clarifies its highly interesting image.

The basic theme in Lycopodium has to do with cowardice. Inside, Lycopodium patients are constantly contending with cowardice—moral, social, and physical. They feel themselves to be weak and inadequate, incapable of fulfilling their responsibilities in life, and so they avoid responsibilities. Externally, however, the Lycopodium patient may present to the world an image of capability, extroverted friendliness, and courage, which can make the true image of the remedy difficult to perceive without skillful probing on the part of the homeopath.

The central area in which Lycopodium shows itself in early stages is in relationship to sex. The Lycopodium patient seeks situations in which the desire for sexual gratification can be satisfied without having to face the personal responsibilities which are implicit in such intimacy. It is commonly observed in such patients that there has been a long history of one-night stands, in which the patient seeks satisfaction and then walks away without further responsibility. If a sexual partner shows interest in marriage, the Lycopodium patient becomes fearful of the responsibilities and whether he will be able to fulfill them. Usually, he will leave before becoming "penned in" by the responsibilities of marriage, children, or even other forms of commitment in life.

This relationship to sex is a superficial one. Gratification is the primary motivation; he wants it quick, easy, effortlessly, and without consequences. If such a patient meets a secretary who is by chance alone in an office, the first thought on his mind will be that this is a sexual opportunity, and he will likely make advances. Such patients may also visit prostitutes frequently, as this contact implies no responsibilities. It is not as if the Lycopodium patient's desire is so intense, as it is in Platina; the Lycopodium constitution is too weak for such intensity, but when the desire does arise, the Lycopodium way of handling it is focused on the superficial gratification of the moment and the avoidance of responsibility.

Once married, the Lycopodium man or woman may well experience sexual dysfunctions because of the fear of being unable to fulfill the responsibilities of intimacy. The woman may be unable to have orgasm, or the man may experience impotence in the form of either premature ejaculation or absence of erection. Internally, the Lycopodium patient feels a deep state of inadequacy and weakness, and this is challenged most noticeably in the intimate marriage relationship. The Lycopodium patient, sensing this feeling of inadequacy, usually presents a strong, courageous, competent image to the world, but his bluff is called when responsibility and performance are required, as in marriage. So, it is in the marriage situation where the administration of Lycopodium can have some of the most gratifying results.

Such patients are in constant fear that others will discover the truth about their inner state of weakness. They are constantly worried about what others think of them.

Because Lycopodium fits highly intelligent and intellectual people, it is found frequently in professions requiring public performance—priests, lawyers, schoolteachers, even politicians. A priest may feel perfectly well before giving a sermon, but upon reaching the pulpit and realizing that so many eyes are upon him, he may suddenly suffer gastritis pain or great anxiety. Such a person may be able to carry out the task properly, but very often the physical or emotional suffering will seriously interfere with functioning. Again, this situation is a manifestation of anxiety in the face of responsibility, and the patient may well attempt to escape from his profession, sometimes seeming to use the physical illness as an excuse.

Lycopodium patients may go overboard in presenting a bluff to compensate for the inner feeling of inferiority. They may exaggerate their attainments, their capacities, the people they know. They may go so far as to tell outrageous lies which cannot be supported when the moment comes to produce results. This bloating of their ego-presentation is a compensation for the presumed state of weakness inside, and it is based upon a powerful need to receive admiration and respect from others in order to "prove" themselves.

Eventually, the Lycopodium patient may end up becoming a loner—a spinster or a celibate spiritual seeker. By attempting to avoid responsibility and gain a measure of control over the desire for instant gratification, the patient may decide to become celibate. This is a fragile state of celibacy, however, because the Lycopodium patient is now constantly obsessed even more strongly by sexual thoughts. After years of discipline, the most pious celibate may break down with surprising ease once an opportunity is presented, only to immediately return to the disciplined state later.

With time, the desire for gratification in sex may be replaced by the desire for power. Lycopodium is the only remedy listed under the rubric Love of Power. This clearly is a further attempt to compensate for the inner sense of weakness. This may manifest as a desire for power in the realm of politics or business, but it can also be seen as the desire for spiritual power in spiritual seekers. It is an attempt to acquire power in order to replace the lack of inner strength.

In the second stage of development of Lycopodium pathology, the external bluff becomes even more exaggerated. The patient becomes dictatorial and tyrannical with those around who can be controlled. Lycopodium patients may be timid and passive with co-workers on the job who are not under their control, but become despots at home. A mother may be sweet to her neighbors but tyrannical with her children. By exerting power over others, such people attempt to generate their sense of personal power, just as they previously attempted to bolster their sense of power by seeking the admiration of others through lies and exaggerations.

It is also in the second stage that the Lycopodium cowardice becomes more intense. At this stage, many fears become evident. Lycopodium can become terrified by almost anything—being alone, the dark, ghosts, even strange dogs. It is because of such fears that Lycopodium patients, while basically loners because of their fear of facing responsibility, are said to desire company, but in the next room. There is a great fear of suffering of any kind; thus the Lycopodium patient can become anxious about health to the point of hypochondriasis. The fears and anxieties affect mostly the gastrointestinal tract.

In the third stage, prolonged dissipation of energy, either in the search for sexual gratification or in struggling with the attempt to control it through celibacy, finally results in a deterioration of mental functions. This may begin initially as a confusion or poor memory in the morning, and gradually progresses to a more marked memory loss and intellectual weakness. Finally, the patient degenerates into a state of imbecility or senility. Such patients are likely to end up in rest homes at a relatively early age.

On the physical level, the Lycopodium appearance is fairly distinctive. There is an emaciation of the face, neck, and upper torso. The tissues seem to waste away in these regions, while an excess of fat may accumulate around the abdomen, the hips, and lower limbs. The face tends to be excessively wrinkled, particularly in patterns reflecting the prolonged anxiety and concern Lycopodiums have over what others think of them. The hair may become gray at an early age, and the person may appear considerably older than his actual age. The flapping of the alae nasi (outer boundaries of the nostrils), which is described so frequently in books, is rarely seen in actual practice, because it is mostly limited to acute illness involving dyspnea (labored breathing).

The primary region of action of Lycopodium centers on the genitals, the urinary tract, the gastrointestinal system, and the liver—including complaints such as impotence, frigidity, nephritis, peptic ulcer, colitis, hemorrhoids, and liver disorders. The gastrointestinal tract, in particular, represents the qualities seen throughout Lycopodium.

Just as there is a bloating of the ego-presentation in compensation for the inner sense of weakness, there is also a bloating of the intestines in reaction to weak digestion. The patient is "full of wind" and suffers severely after eating. Also, just as there is an emphasis on superficial gratification in sex, the Lycopodium patient seeks gratification of the palate by craving foods according to their taste—especially sweets and oysters. This comparison extends even further: the Lycopodium patient feels empty and unsatisfied after coition, and suffers excessively after indulging in a meal based on gratification of taste. Lycopodium patients are constantly trying to control their desire for such indulgence.

The weakness of digestion is frequently a consequence of a liver ailment. Lycopodium is often indicated in liver dysfunctions, and it is interesting to note that the liver is commonly associated with mental disturbances which fit the Lycopodium image.

Lycopodium can be compared with many remedies, of course. The anticipatory anxiety which causes such suffering during public functions in Lycopodium can be compared to Gelsemium; in Lycopodium, it refers more to the state of suffering which occurs during the actual task, while Gelsemium is indicated more for the anxiety and symptoms which occur hours and days prior to the task. Silica is a remedy which has a lack of self-confidence, but it suffers mostly from the inability to cope with any circumstance, not only the social and moral responsibilities which concern Lycopodium. Calcacea can have many similarities to Lycopodium but does not have the characteristic cowardice. Natrum muriaticum is also a remedy which presents an outer image in compensation for an inner weakness; but the Natrum muriaticum inner state is one of emotional and sentimental vulnerability rather than the sense of inadequacy felt by Lycopodium.

NATRUM MURIATICUM

The primary characteristic underlying the Natrum muriaticum pathology is *introversion* arising out of a feeling of great vulnerability to emotional injury. Natrum muriaticum patients are emotionally very sensitive; they experience the emotional pain of others, and feel that any form of rejection, ridicule, humiliation, or grief would be personally intolerable. Consequently, they create a wall of invulnerability, become enclosed in their own worlds, and prefer to maintain control over their circumstances. They avoid being hurt at all costs.

People susceptible to developing the Natrum muriaticum type of pathology are emotionally sensitive and vulnerable, but quite clear and strong on mental and physical levels. Mentally, they have a high degree of objectivity and awareness, as well as a great sense of responsibility. For this reason, they are likely to be the sympathetic ear to whom others turn when distressed. The emotional sensitivity and the sense of responsibility readily lead such people into fields of counselling, psychotherapy, the ministry, etc. While listening sympathetically to someone else's suffering, such people maintain their objectivity and appear to be very strong. They internally absorb the pain of others, however, and they dwell on it later; particularly, they wonder, "How would I react in such a situation? Would I be able to take it?"

Throughout life, individuals with Natrum muriaticum tendencies experience deeply all impressions of life, accumulating awareness and understanding beyond their age. They are strong and enjoy being presented with challenging circumstances, even those involving emotional risk. At first, they enjoy company and thrive on the nourishment of emotional contact with others. They enjoy receiving affection from others—indeed, they inwardly expect and demand it—even though they do not themselves express affection easily. They are so sensitive that they feel hurt by the slightest comment or gesture that might imply ridicule or rejection. Natrum muriaticum adolescents, for example, are reluctant to date, for fear of rejection. Even imagined slights can cause suffering. After being hurt several times, they learn to become cautious. They will think twice before becoming involved in an emotional experience. They turn to introverted activities which are emotionally "safe"—i.e., reading books (usually romantic fiction or things having practical value in human relations), listening to music, dwelling on ideas and fantasies.

They can become quite content in their isolation. They tend to be self-contained, desiring to solve problems by themselves without trusting help from other people. Gradually, they come to the point of not needing contact with the outside world. If someone intrudes upon their private, introverted world, they may feel resentful. Their primary concern in life becomes, "not to hurt and not to be hurt."

The issue of emotional pain, in themselves or in others, is important to such people. Just as personal humiliation would be the end of the world for them, they are completely incapable of knowingly inflicting pain on others. For this reason, they become very serious. They cannot make jokes that might inadvertently ridicule someone else. They may appear cold and overly objective to others because they are so intent on not revealing their own emotional vulnerability or creating injury to others. This, combined with the Natrum muriaticum sense of responsibility, results in guilt being a strong motivating factor in the lives of such people.

Physically, children with Natrum muriaticum tendencies are likely to be thin and delicate. It is common to see a fine, precise horizontal line dividing the lower eyelid in two. This line is commonly seen in young girls with hysterical personalities; other remedies showing this line include Asafoetida, Lilium tigrinum, and Moschus. In addition, there may be a characteristic crack in the middle of the lower lip.

A Natrum muriaticum child is very sensitive to disharmony. If the parents fight, the child may not react immediately but will suffer inside, perhaps even to the point of acquiring a physical ailment. These children are usually quite well-behaved; it is not necessary to severely discipline them because a mere glance conveying disapproval will suffice.

The hysterical tendency in Natrum muriaticum children is seen readily when they are severely reprimanded. They then react to an extreme degree, falling on the floor in a tantrum, kicking and screaming. Consolation or reassurance are of no avail, and may actually make them worse; they will continue with the tantrum until they themselves decide to stop.

At an older age, the hysterical tendency shows itself in another way. Ordinarily, Natrum muriaticum people do not express emotion readily; they do not cry easily, for example, when suffering a grief. They may be quite serious in their demeanor. However, when nervous or under stress, they tend to laugh over serious matters, then to giggle hysterically; as this giggling becomes uncontrollable, it dissolves into hysterical weeping.

Adolescents of this type are likely to be quiet and withdrawn, but with a sense of responsibility and integrity. At a party, they tend to sit on the sidelines, enjoying themselves by watching others and imagining what they are experiencing. If they are attracted to someone, they will not be flirtatious or friendly. Indeed, they may appear to pay no attention at all, only watching the other out of the corner of the eye. They are liable to fantasize that the other person is likewise attracted, and they may romantically blow the entire situation out of proportion.

This is the reason why Kent states that a young girl who needs Natrum muriaticum will easily fall in love with a married man, or someone unattainable. This then causes intense anguish and grief, and the result is an even greater introversion.

They develop intense emotional and sentimental attachments for people, but they do not show their feelings. A daughter may have a deep feeling for her father without anyone else realizing it. Then the father dies. The daughter grieves silently, locking herself in her room and crying in her pillow. To the surprise of everyone around her who did not realize the depth of her affection, she becomes very introverted, desiring only to be alone with her books and her music. There is no moaning or crying in front of others—merely occasional sighing perhaps. This internal state continues until she finally breaks down. Then there is uncontrolled, hysterical sobbing with massive shaking of the body, spasms, and twitchings. Such an outburst usually lasts just a short time, and she quickly regains control and composure.

The first stage of pathology in Natrum muriaticum appears on the physical level. There may be gastritis, arthritis, migraine headaches, canker sores, or herpes on the lower lip. As might be expected, such conditions are likely to occur after a period of introversion following a severe grief or humiliation.

Alternatively, the patient may become hysterically reactive to every influence in the environment—overly sensitive to noise, to light, to cigarette smoke, etc. In such patients, allergies and eczema are common.

Neurological disorders are also very common in Natrum muriaticum. Neuralgias affecting the left eye or the left intercostal nerves, for example, are frequent. Multiple sclerosis often responds to Natrum muriaticum as well, when the totality of symptoms fits. Heart disease can occur, but it tends to manifest as arrhythmias and palpitations—which arise from the influence of the nervous system on the heart.

It is during the earliest phases of pathology that some of the most well-known Natrum muriaticum keynotes are found. The patient has a strong desire for salt, and an aversion to slimy food and to fat; there is an aversion to chicken as well. Characteristically, there is an intolerance to heat, sensitivity to light, and aggravation (of headaches and skin particularly) from the sun. These are true to varying degrees in all of the Natrums, but they are more or less equally expressed in Natrum muriaticum. The Natrum muriaticum aggravations from sun and light are not as marked as they are in Natrum sulphuricum, and its aggravation from the sun is not as marked as in Natrum carbonicum. The Natrum muriaticum patient may be sensitive to both heat and to cold, though usually more so to heat. It is less sensitive to heat than Natrum sulphuricum, and also less sensitive to cold than Natrum carbonicum.

A characteristic symptom of Natrum muriaticum is the inability to pass urine or stool in the presence of others. This arises from the fear of ridicule, resulting in a chronic tension of sphincter muscles which can be relaxed only in private.

As the emotional vulnerability becomes increasingly pathological, the patient becomes depressed. This is a depression which is inconsolable, and may even become suicidal. Suppose, for example, a young man experiences a severe rejection or grief; he retires to his room and puts on the saddest music he can find. The music is not designed to alleviate the depression, but rather to add to it. He wallows in depression. If one thing has gone wrong, he exaggerates everything out of all proportion, imagining that every aspect of his life is cause for despair. He allows no one to help; he tries to solve the problem within himself. Eventually, when the depression begins to pass, he regains a more appropriate perspective on life, and music will at that point relieve the remnants of the depression. It is in this sense that music may be either aggravating or ameliorating to Natrum muriaticum, depending on the circumstances.

This kind of depression is a kind of hysterical reaction. Ordinarily, the Natrum muriaticum patient is objective as long as control over the emotions is maintained; but when emotional control breaks down, the patient becomes irrational, and the emotional sphere rules everything.

As the pathology moves beyond the phase of depression, the patient begins to experience periodicity of physical symptoms and alternation of moods.

Physical complaints occur at predictable intervals and times. This is why Natrum muriaticum is often indicated in patients who have suffered from malaria in the past or who have been adversely affected by quinine drugs; it also can be useful in patients in whose family there has been malaria. Migraine attacks often seen in Natrum muriaticum patients tend to occur at fixed times, usually between 10 a.m. and 3 p.m. Asthmatic attacks, likewise, tend to occur between 5–7 p.m.

The moods swing from unreasonable depression to unreasonable exhilaration. As the patient's objectivity becomes interfered with, everything on the emotional level is carried to extremes.

By this stage, some of the characteristic physical symptoms may gradually disappear. As the pathology progresses to deeper levels, there may no longer be desire for salt, aversion to slimy or fatty foods, aggravation from the sun, etc. The disappearance of these traits is directly proportional to the progressive deepening of the pathological state. Often it will be necessary for the homeopath to inquire into such symptoms not only in the present, but also the past.

As the pathology begins to reach into the emotional level, the first fear that develops is claustrophobia. In early stages, Natrum muriaticum patients enjoy relative emotional freedom and resent any constrictions imposed by others. Later on, their own vulnerability causes them to close off. When they perceive the same kind of enclosure outside themselves (i.e., closed or narrow places) as they have created within, they become fearful.

Along with the claustrophobia, there occurs a rigidification of the emotional and mental planes. The patient develops fixed ideas; things are seen in terms of good or bad, right or wrong, correct or incorrect, practical or impractical.

Eventually, a hypochondriacal anxiety about health emerges, particularly in regard to heart disease. This hypochondriasis is related to the fastidiousness seen in Natrum muriaticum. The patient is driven by a compulsive need to avoid contamination—always cleaning, washing hands, disinfecting everything. In Natrum muriaticum, fastidiousness is specifically a fear of microbial contamination, and not so much the feeling of *disgust* seen in other remedies (Sulphur, Pulsatilla, Mercury, Phosphorus, Mezereum). Also, in Natrum muriaticum, anxiety about health is much less significant than hypochondriasis, which is more of an anxiety-less compulsive attention to details about health.

Finally, even the compulsive control mechanisms break down completely, and the person openly expresses everything which previously had been disallowed. They become shameless, exhibitionistic, speak in obscenities, etc. In the final stage, Natrum muriaticum patients do not usually lose mental control to the point of developing full-blown insanity, but shameless behavior may occur.

Natrum muriaticum is such a deep-acting remedy, and it is so commonly indicated in our Western World, that there are many other remedies to which it should be compared.

Ignatia, of course, is the closest of all remedies to Natrum muriaticum. In many respects, they are virtually identical. For this reason, they often replace one another in particular cases. Generally, Ignatia acts more superficially and is more likely to be indicated in cases where patients' reactions are more superficial. Natrum muriaticum patients have greater strength; they can tolerate more emotional stress and more intense shocks without breaking down. In Ignatia, the person breaks down with relatively minor stress. In addition, the Ignatia pathology does not as readily affect the physical level. Thus, Ignatia is more indicated in emotional reactions appearing after ordinary griefs experienced in life, whereas Natrum muriaticum is more commonly indicated in instances of extraordinary stresses, particularly those causing breakdown on the physical level.

The Ignatia patient frequently feels constricted in the throat or in breathing, especially following an emotional shock. The characteristic Ignatia sighing is an attempt to relieve this sensation of constriction. Ignatia cries more easily and is more likely to cry during the homeopathic interview than Natrum muriaticum. Following a grief, the Ignatia patient is less likely to experience sleeplessness than Natrum muriaticum.

Frequently, particularly when there are mostly physical symptoms, Phosphorus may be difficult to differentiate from Natrum muriaticum. Physically, both look quite similar—thin, sensitive, even perhaps hyperthyroid. The main point of differentiation, of course, is whether the patient has a personality which is closed or open. The sensitive person who tends to be more withheld and eva-sive, who leans back in the chair while describing symp-toms, is more likely to need Natrum muriaticum. The Phosphorus patient, on the other hand, is very open and expressive of emotion, tending to lean forward and engage the interviewer in personal contact.

Lilium tigrinum is a highly hysterical remedy, as is Natrum muriaticum. If a Lilium tigrinum patient experi-ences rejection or humiliation, however, there is an in-stantaneous, impulsive reaction; the Natrum muriaticum patient, on the other hand, will suffer inside and wait quite a long time before finally breaking down into a hysterical reaction. Lilium tigrinum is also more likely to be malicious and cruel during such a reaction, whereas the Natrum muriaticum person would rather inflict suffering on himself than cause pain to anyone else.

Moschus is another hysterical remedy, but the differen-tiation is quite easy. This type of hysteria is designed for others to observe. It is manipulative, an attempt to emo-tionally blackmail others into a desired response. Natrum muriaticum would rather hide any reaction as much as possible.

Pulsatilla is sometimes confused with Natrum muriati-cum. Both are intolerant to heat, aggravated in the sun, and averse to fat. Pulsatilla, however, is emotionally highly expressive, automatically giving of affection. When a Pul-satilla patient cries (which occurs easily), it is a "sweet," gentle crying, whereas the Natrum muriaticum weeping is a spasmodic, loud sobbing which wracks the whole body. Pulsatilla patients that are suffering will actively seek help from others and depend on them; Natrum muriaticum is more self-reliant, preferring to solve problems by themselves.

Lycopodium is a remedy which displays an outer shell created in reaction to an inner state, but internally it is weak and cowardly. Natrum muriaticum is strong, but emotionally vulnerable to being hurt.

Sepia is closely related to Natrum muriaticum. Particularly in children, they may be very difficult to tell apart. Sepia children are very sensitive, and much more excitable than Natrum muriaticum. In their excitability, they can become flushed and hyperactive. In adulthood, it is as if the Sepia patient has been broken down by this excessive excitability, becoming fatigued, mentally dulled, and apathetic. Natrum muriaticum feels affection but does not express it easily; Sepia fundamentally has lost it. The Sepia patient is much more likely to be malicious and cruel, almost enjoying hurting others; this would be unthinkable for Natrum muriaticum.

PHOSPHORUS

Diffusion is the theme which runs through the Phosphorus pathology. Diffusion is the process of spreading outward into the environment, like smoke spreading outward into the air, or the color from a tea bag diffusing uniformly into water. The same happens to the energy, the awareness, the emotions, and even the blood of the Phosphorus patient. It is as if there are no barriers for this—physical, emotional, or mental. Because of this, the Phosphorus patient is vulnerable to all types of influences. On the physical level, we see that almost any injury or stress results in hemorrhage; this occurs because the sheaths of the blood vessels are weak and easily allow the blood to diffuse into surrounding tissues. On the emotional plane, the Phosphorus patient's emotions freely go out toward others, with little ability of the patient to contain them and protect the self from emotional vulnerability. Mentally, the patient easily forgets himself, even to the degree that awareness can become too diffuse and unfocused; the patient becomes easily "spaced out."

Let us first describe a person in the healthy state who nevertheless possesses the Phosphorus predilection, which can emerge into a disease state if the defense mechanism becomes overwhelmed by too much stress; in doing so, however, keep in mind that we only prescribe on the pathological symptoms, not on the healthy ones. The Phosphorus patient physically is usually lean, tall, and delicate in features, hair, skin, and hands. As a child, this person is warm, outgoing, affectionate, artistic or musical, and very sensitive. The child is very open and *impressionable*; one can "see through" such a child, whose being is effortlessly manifested, without much reserve. During adolescence, there is a tremendous growth spurt which leads to the typically lean, lanky appearance.

Throughout life, the Phosphorus type person is a warm, friendly, extrovert who enjoys friendship and company very much, but also may enjoy solitude to pursue artistic endeavors. Such a person is enjoyable to have around, because he or she is truly sympathetic, freely putting the interest of friends above personal concerns. The Phosphorus person is highly intelligent and refined. There are no secrets for such a person; whatever is on his mind he shares freely. Warmth and affection diffuse freely toward friends, and even strangers. Much of his or her life revolves around interpersonal relationships. Such a person makes a good politician, the type that pushes for humanitarian causes, or a Phosphorus type may become a sales agent because he has the ability to sell anything he believes in.

The Phosphorus person is very impressionable and will believe anything which is told to him in an area outside of his own competence; then, once he has adopted a belief, he will be enthusiastic and convincing to others.

Such a person makes an enjoyable patient for the homeopath because he is impressionable and trusting; the Phosphorus patient believes in what the prescriber tells him and follows directions willingly and with effusive gratitude. Right from the first interview, the patient views the prescriber as a friend, shaking his hand warmly, sitting forward on the seat, and perhaps reaching out to touch the prescriber's hand or wrist when emphasizing a point. This patient gives symptoms freely, without holding back. There is a predisposition toward anxieties of various types, but these are relieved easily by just a few reassuring words.

The diffusion of awareness is evident by the fact that the Phosphorus patient is easily startled. All of us can relate to the state of mind of daydreaming; awareness drifts to a far-off place or circumstance. During a daydream, if there is a sudden noise, like a blaring horn, a slamming door, or a burst of thunder, the daydreamer is startled because awareness is pulled suddenly and joltingly back into the immense reality. This is the state to which the Phosphorus patient is highly susceptible. It is a diffusion of awareness which the patient may not be able to control readily. During a thunderstorm, the normal person will hear a clap of thunder and then easily prepare himself for more; the Phosphorus patient, however, tends to become diffuse automatically, and so will be startled with each noise.

In the first stage of Phosphorus pathology, the physical symptoms usually predominate. In the childish stage of development (whether 5 years or 35 years of age), there may be a tendency to easy hemorrhages. Nosebleeds occur

with little provocation. Menses may be profuse and prolonged. The bleeding tends to be bright red in color. The
bleeding tendency is symbolic of the general essence of
Phosphorus. What warmth and brightness the Phosphorus
patient possesses diffuse freely outward, with little sense of
barriers.

It is at this stage that we see the Phosphorus patient
who is easily refreshed by sleep. This is understandable
when we reflect that sleep is a time when the ordinary
effort to maintain immediate physical awareness is relaxed
and rested. People who are more controlled and mental-
ized take a long time to achieve this rest; they must fall
into a deep sleep. The Phosphorus patient, on the other
hand, is quickly refreshed because his awareness can diffuse
in this manner very readily.

During this stage, we also see the characteristic Phosphorus thirst, particularly for cold drinks. If there happens to be burning in the stomach (Phosphorus experiences
burning pains internally—a manifestation of warmth), the
pains will be relieved by cold things; but this lasts only
until the drink or food warms in the stomach, and then
the stomach may be again aggravated. There is a typical
craving for salt; both the thirst and the craving for salt
may well signify an imbalance of electrolytes in the body,
of which phosphates are one. There is a craving for fish,
which again we can surmise to be related to a lack of
phosphorus in the system. In addition, Phosphorus has a
craving for chocolate and sweets. Considering the thirst
and the craving for sweets, it is easy to see the Phosphorus
predilection for diabetes.

As the physical pathology progresses further, the process
of hemorrhage may be evident on deeper levels. There may
be painless hemorrhage from the gastrointestinal tract,
resulting in an unexpected hematemesis or melena. There

may be bronchitis in an early and mild phase, yet with hemoptysis of bright red blood. There may be hematuria unaccompanied by any other symptoms. Laboratory tests and X-rays may be done, and nothing found. In these circumstances, think of Phosphorus as a possible remedy.

While the physical symptoms predominate, there are few symptoms in the emotional or mental spheres. As the pathology progresses, however, into the second stage, we see a subsidence of the physical symptoms and an increase in anxieties and fears. Of course, there is a strong anxiety about others. In Phosphorus, this is a true anxiety for the welfare of another, whether friend or stranger. It can be carried to a pathological degree of anxiety, dissipating even the energy of the patient himself. This is the true state of sympathy, whereas other remedies in the same rubric are anxious about others out of a primary motive of self-concern.

There is a strong anxiety about health in Phosphorus. The patient becomes so suggestible that even if he hears of someone else with a particular illness, he will be concerned about the possibility that he also might have that illness. This vulnerability to suggestion, however, is easily assuaged by counter-suggestion; a few reassuring words by the homeopath, and the patient sighs with relief and is profusely thankful, only to come back when he hears another alarming possibility.

It is during this stage that there is the emergence of many fears. There is fear of the dark, fear of being alone, and fear at twilight. There may be a fear of thunderstorms. At first these anxieties and fears are fairly mild, and still corroborated by thirst and refreshed sleep.

As the third stage emerges, the patient becomes overwhelmed by the anxieties and fears. Whereas before they were mild and manageable by simple reassurance, they gradually occupy more and more of the energy and attention of the patient. The patient finds it increasingly difficult to relax, and anxiety may lead to hyperventilation and resultant imbalances in the pH of the blood. The undercurrent of anxiety and tension prevent relaxation even during sleep; the patient begins to experience unrefreshing sleep. The patient awakes unrefreshed, and also with great anxiety (like Lachesis, Graphites, and Arsenicum).

Eventually, the continuous anxiety becomes a "free-floating anxiety" with no identifiable cause. There is a fear that something bad will happen which pervades the person's life, like background music. Every possibility is anticipated with fear. There is a fear of impending disease, particularly a fear of cancer (rather than heart disease), but eventually the fear of *any* impending disease.

Finally, the Phosphorus patient falls into a fear of death, a panic state over the idea that death is imminent. The patient feels like he is dying, especially when he is alone. There is the sensation of fuzziness internally, like bubbles rising and diffusing outward, or that the soul is leaving the body. There is great panic, hyperventilation, excitability, and palpitations. This is the point when the patient develops a need for company, because of the fear that death is imminent. The need for company can be so strong as to drive him to leave his house to find friends to talk to. This is not a need to talk to people about his health in particular, as in Arsenicum; rather, Phosphorus just feels the need to talk to anybody about anything, in order to relieve the panic.

As the states of fear increase, many of the other corroborating symptoms on the physical level disappear. There may be no thirst, no craving for salt, and no craving for fish.

Finally, in the fourth stage, the mind breaks down completely. The fears diminish, but the mind degenerates. There is a difficulty in concentration, an inability to think coherently, or an inability to understand what is being said by others. The body and the mind become weak. The patient becomes indifferent to company, and indifferent to surroundings. The result is a state of senility or imbecility. Another common end result in Phosphorus is a stroke in which many mental faculties are lost.

This final stage can be a very difficult one in which to prescribe, because there is a paucity of symptoms to distinguish Phosphorus from other remedies. For this reason, a careful history of the past sequence of events and a proper knowledge of the stages of pathology of remedies is crucial to being able to benefit the patient.

Once the essence of Phosphorus is seen, one needs only to confirm the remedy with corroborating symptons. From experience, some of the most useful are: thirst, desire for salt, desire for fish, desire for chocolate, desire for sweets, worse left side, unable to sleep on the left side, formication of the tips of the fingers, painless loss of voice. In addition, different Phosphorus patients may be either warmblooded or chilly—though not in the same patient.

Bibliography

Allen, Dr. H. C. *Keynotes and Characteristics.*
——— *Materia Medica of Nosodes.*
Allen, Dr. J. H. *Chronic Miasms, Psora and Sycosis.*
——— *Diseases and Therapeutics of the Skin.*
Allen, Dr. T. F. *A Primer of Materia Medica.*
——— *A Hand Book of Materia Medica and Homoeo-Therapeutics.*
Banerjee, Dr. N. K. *Notes on Cholera by Hahnemann and Others.*
——— *Spirit of Homoeopathy.*
Banerjee, Dr. P. N. *Chronic Disease and Its Cause and Cure.*
Berne, A. *What Is Homoeopathic Dilution and How Homoeopathic Medicine Acts.*
Blackwood, Dr. A. L. *Materia Medica. Therapeutics.*
Boenninghausen, Dr. Von. *Intermittent Fever.*
——— *Therapeutic Pocket Book.*
——— *Sides of the Body.*
——— *Lesser Writings.*
——— *Characteristic and Reportory.*

Boericke, Dr. Wm. *Materia Medica with Reportory.*

Boericke, Dr. Garth. *Principles of Homoeopathy.*

Boericke and Dewey, Drs. *Twelve Tissue Remedies of Schuessler.*

Boger, Dr. C. M. *Synoptic Key to Materia Medica.*

———— *The Study of Materia Medica.*

———— *The Study of Materia Medica and Taking the Case.*

———— *Times of Remedies and Moon Phases.*

———— *Philosophy of Healing.*

Borland, Dr. Douglas. *Children Types.*

Boyd, Dr. Linn. *A Study of the Simile in Medicine.*

Bradford, Dr. T. H. *Life and Letters of Dr. S. Hahnemann.*

Burnett, Dr. J. C. *Curability of Cataract.*

———— *Fifty Reasons for Being a Homoeopath.*

———— *Cure for Consumption.*

———— *Delicate, Backward Children.*

———— *Diseases of the Skin.*

Clarke, Dr. J. H. *Dictionary of Materia Medica.*

———— *Prescriber.*

Close, Dr. S. *Genius of Homoeopathy.*

———— *Philosophy.*

Cowperthwaite. *Text Book of Materia Medica and Therapeutics.*

Dewey, Dr. W. A. *Essentials of Homoeo Materia Medica.*

———— *Practical Homoeo Therapeutics.*

———— *Essentials of Therapeutics.*

Dudgeon, Dr. R. E. *Hahnemann's Therapeutic Hints.*

———— *Hahnemann's Organon.*

Duham, Dr. C. *Materia Medica.*

———— *Therapeutics.*

Farrington, Dr. E. A. *Clinical Materia Medica.*

———— *Comparisons in Materia Medica with Therapeutic Hints.*

———— *Lesser Writings.*

Five Doctors. *Why I Became a Homoeopath.*

Gross, Dr. H. *Comparative Materia Medica.*

Guernsey, Dr. H. N. *Keynotes to Materia Medica.*

———— *Avoided Subjects.*

Guernsey, Dr. W. J. *Desires and Aversions.*

Hahnemann, Dr. Samuel. *Organon of Medicine*, translated by Wm. Boericke.

———— *Organon of Medicine*, translated by R. Dudgeon.

———— *Chronic Diseases.*

———— *Spirit of Homoeopathy.*

———— *Therapeutic Hints.*

———— *Materia Medica Pura.*

Hempel, Dr. J. C. *Science of Homoeopathy.*

Hering, Dr. C. *Domestic Physician.*

———— *Condensed Materia Medica.*

———— *Guiding Symptoms* (10 Vols.)

Holcombe, Dr. A. W. *Spasms and Convulsions.*

Holcombe, Dr. W. H. *How I Became a Homoeopath and the Truth about Homoeopathy.*

Homoeopathic Pharmacopoeia (U.S.A.). Published by the American Institute of Homoeopathy.

Hughes, Dr. R. *Principles and Practice of Homoeopathy.*

———— *Manual of Pharmacodynamics.*

Jahr, Dr. G. H. G. *Diseases of Females and Infants on Breast.*

———— *Venereal Diseases.*

———— *Forty Years Practice.*

Johnson, Dr. I. D. *A Guide to Homoeopathic Practice.*

———— *Therapeutic Key.*

Kent, Dr. J. T. *Lectures on Homoeopathic Materia Medica.*

———— *New Remedies.*

——— *Repertory.*

——— *What the Doctor Needs to Know for Successful Prescriptions.*

——— *Lectures on Homoeopathic Philosophy.*

Knerr, C. V. *Drug Relationship.*

——— *Reportory.*

Lippe, Dr. Ad. *Keynotes to Materia Medica.*

——— *Materia Medica.*

Lippe, Dr. C. *Reportory.*

Nash, Dr. E. B. *How to Take the Case.*

——— *Leaders in Homoeopathic Therapeutics.*

——— *Leaders in Typhoid Fever.*

——— *Regional Leaders.*

——— *The Testimony of the Clinic.*

——— *Sulphur.*

——— *Leaders in Respiratory Organs.*

Paracelsus. *Selected Writings*, ed. by Jolande Jacobi, Pantheon Books.

Pierce, Dr. W. L. *Plain Talks on Materia Medica.*

Pulford, Drs. A. and D. T. *Key to Materia Medica.*

——— *Materia Medica of Graphic Drug Pictures.*

——— *Leaders in Pneumonia.*

Robert, Dr. H. A. *The Principles and Art of Cure.*

——— *Sensations As If.*

Roy, Dr. C. K. *Etiology in Homoeopathy.*

Royal, Dr. George. *Materia Medica.*

——— *Handy Book of Reference.*

Ruddock, Dr. E. H. *Stepping Stone to Homoeopathy.*

Schuessler, Dr. M. *An Abridged Therapy.*

——— *Manual for Bio-chemical Treatment of Diseases.*

——— *The Tissue Remedies.*

Shepherd, Dr. Dorothy. *Magic of the Minimum Dose.*

——— *More Magic of the Minimum Dose.*

———— *First Aider.*
Vannier, Dr. L. *Difficult and Backward Children.*
———— *Human Medicine.*
Weir, Sir John. *Science and Art of Homoeopathy.*
Wheeler, Dr. C. E. *Principle and Practice of Homoe-opathy.*
Wright, Elizabeth. *Brief Study Course in Homoeopathy.*

APPENDIX III

Resources

Homeopathic Pharmacies
(where books listed in the Bibliography may be obtained)

Ainsworths
Homeopathic Pharmacy
38 New Cavendish Street
London W1M 7LH
ENGLAND

Nelson's Pharmacy
73 Duke Street, Grosvenor Square
London W1M 6BY
ENGLAND

Boericke and Tafel
1011 Arch Street
Philadelphia, PA 19107
USA

Luyties Pharmacal Company
4200 Laclede Avenue
St. Louis, MO 63108
USA

Humphreys Pharmacal, Inc.
63 Meadow Rd.
Rutherford, NJ 07070
USA

International Organizations

International Foundation for the Promotion of
    Homeopathy
President, George Vithoulkas
76 Lee Street
Mill Valley, CA 94941
USA

International Homeopathic League
President, C. Eenhorn
Bloemendaal, Bloemendaalseweg 17
Les Pays-Bas
Amsterdam
HOLLAND

National Organizations

National Center for Homeopathy
6231 Leesburg Pike, Suite 506
Falls Church, VA 22044
Telephone: 202-534-4363
USA

INDEX